PSYCHOANALYSIS

Evolution
and
Development

PSYCHOANALYSIS

Clara Thompson

With a new introduction by
Paul Roazen

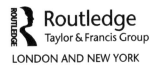

Routledge
Taylor & Francis Group

LONDON AND NEW YORK

Originally published in 1950 by Thomas Nelson & Sons.

Published 2003 by Transaction Publishers

Published 2017 by Routledge
2 Park Square, Milton Park, Abingdon, Oxon, OX14 4RN
711 Third Avenue, New York, NY 10017, USA

Routledge is an imprint of the Taylor & Francis Group, an informa business

Library of Congress Catalog Number: 2002073264

Library of Congress Cataloging-in-Publication Data

Thompson, Clara, 1893-1958.
  Psychoanalysis: evolution and development / Clara Thompson ; with a new introduction by Paul Roazen.
     p. cm.
  Includes bibliographical references and index.
  ISBN 0-7658-0967-2 (alk. paper)
    1. Psychoanalysis—History. I. Title.

BF175.T45 2002
150.19'5—dc21   2002073264

ISBN 13: 978-0-7658-0967-4 (pbk)

To the memory of Henry Major

CONTENTS

INTRODUCTION TO THE TRANSACTION EDITION

CLARA THOMPSON WAS A LEADING REPRESENTATIVE OF the cultural interpersonal school of psychoanalysis, sometimes known as the "neo-Freudians." Although psychoanalytic sectarianism once meant that "classical analysts" in the middle of the twentieth century viewed Thompson and her allies with the greatest suspicion and distrust, this innovative group of thinkers succeeded so well that as a movement of theorizing they have virtually disappeared now as a recognizable, separate stream of thought. Unlike their more bureaucratic opponents within the so-called mainstream, the neo-Freudians were relatively egalitarian among themselves and eclectic in how they put their ideas forth. The fanaticism of their opponents meant that the criticism they underwent is easier to recall, along with the various ideological crimes they were accused of promoting, than the spirit of tolerance and catholicity they espoused. Precisely because earlier struggles in the history of psychoanalysis are so easily forgotten today it is worthwhile to memorialize those embattled pioneers who now are so readily neglected, even if the substance of what they once proposed has been widely accepted.

Clara Thompson was born on Oct. 3, 1893 in Providence, Rhode Island. Her parents were both Baptists, and she did her

pre-medical studies at Pembroke, the college for women at
Brown University. She then entered medical school at Johns
Hopkins in 1916. She came in personal contact with William
Alanson White, who was superintendent at St. Elizabeth's Hospi-
tal in Washington, D.C. She did her psychiatric residency un-
der Adolf Meyer at Hopkins, and soon became friendly with
Harry Stack Sullivan, the great pioneer in the psychotherapeu-
tic approach to schizophrenia. She also spent the summers of
1928 and 1929 working with Sandor Ferenczi in Budapest.
Ferenczi had already made some presentations in New York
City, and he was known not only as a great personal favorite of
Freud's but as the analyst with a particular interest in
psychoanalysis's possibilities as a therapeutic agent.

   In 1930 Clara served as the first president of the Washington-
Baltimore Psychoanalytic Society, and in 1931 she left for
Budapest to have an analysis with Ferenczi. (Meyer had been
dead-set against the personal analysis of analysts, a practice that
was just getting underway in the 1920s, and her decision to defy
him earlier for the sake of seeing a Washington analyst meant
her dismissal from Meyer's clinic.) Some patients went with her
from Baltimore, and while in Budapest she had over half a dozen
cases. After Ferenczi's death in 1933, she returned to the States,
where she settled in New York City. She renewed her friendship
with Sullivan, and also met Karen Horney. Soon Erich Fromm
joined them as an ally, and Clara eventually went to him for
another analysis.

   By the late 1930s the American cultural school of interpersonal psychoanalysis was flourishing, and counted among its
members the anthropologist Ruth Benedict as well as the psychiatrist Abram Kardiner. They were reformers who were up-

to-date in their social science, in contrast to Freud who had more of a nineteenth-century armchair approach to the study of society. These "neo-Freudians" were reformers trying to get away, among other objectives, from the ritualistic technical approach of traditional analysts. Looking at Freud's theories in the context of the social characteristics that had marked his own era was one way of breaking free from the dogmatic slumbers of the orthodox psychoanalysis of that day.

When Horney in 1941 was dismissed as a training analyst from the New York Psychoanalytic Society, Clara Thompson resigned with her and a few other faculty members. Along with Fromm and Horney they founded the American Association for the Advancement of Psychoanalysis. Radicals can be hard to hold together, and Horney and Fromm had a falling-out ostensibly over the issue of whether non-medical analysts could be full-fledged members. In 1943 Clara joined with Fromm, and his first-wife Freida Fromm-Reichmann, in creating the New York branch of the William Alanson White Psychiatric Foundation. Sullivan also took part in their work. After a series of illnesses in the mid-1950s, including a malignant polyp that was removed, Clara was diagnosed with cirrhosis of the liver and died Dec. 20, 1958.

Clara Thompson's *Psychoanalysis: Evolution and Development* (1950) remains an enormously fair-minded discussion of the history of psychoanalytic theory and therapy. (It was written with the collaboration of Patrick Mullahy, an Irish-born philosopher who did much to clarify and popularize Sullivan's ideas.) Although she was writing this book before the growth of Freud biographical studies that flourished after the appearance of Ernest Jones's official biography, what she had to say about the history of Freud's school still stands up. She refused to endorse any of the mythology about so-called deviations from the founder of psychoanalysis, and so she could see the pros and cons of the thinking of people like Alfred Adler and Carl G. Jung. And she traced how these dissenting voices fed into the work of later thinkers like Otto Rank, Wilhelm Reich, Horney, and Fromm. Fromm himself, for example, could not always acknowledge his predecessors as readily as someone with Clara Thompson's distance.

Psychoanalysis was a theory of personality as well as a technique of therapy. Since Freud had been born in 1856, and was such an outstanding representative of the culture of old Vienna, Clara thought there was plenty of room for revising classical psychoanalytic thinking in the light of later developments. And such revisionism could take place, she believed, without losing touch with the essential appreciation for the importance of the dynamic unconscious. Freud's biological outlook needed to be supplemented by a more culturally sophisticated orientation, and Clara Thompson was among those who tried to put Freud's libido concepts into historical perspective. For example, this meant that the Oedipus complex was not the universal as described by Freud but a consequence of patriarchal society.

And instead of psychoanalysis having as its objective the release of tensions she proposed that the goal ought to be the growth of the total personality. Further, her revisionism meant that the scope of psychoanalytic treatment could be broadened well beyond the neuroses Freud had sought to explain. As she understood better than most the impact of the social environment on character formation, that meant that the psychology of women needed to be rethought; differences between men and women could be partly explained by the social expectations that traditional Western culture had imposed on them. Psychoanalysis had to beware of incorporating into its treatment setting the dominant patterns of social conformity.

According to Thompson and her allies the whole analyst-patient relationship needed to be reconceptualized; the real personality of the therapist has to be acknowledged, and the full human interplay between client and analyst requires examining. The formalities of classical analysis had had as the central objective the reconstruction of the patient's early childhood, but Clara was insisting on the therapeutic necessity of also understanding the day-to-day real relationship between analyst and patient. Ferenczi had taught that patients need to know realistically that the analyst is not perfect, and have a chance to evaluate the limitations of the analyst.

At the time Clara Thompson first put forward these ideas, it amounted, from the point of view of orthodox analysis, to another heretical assault on Freud's legacy. When Horney, Fromm, Sullivan, and Thompson first put forward their ideas, it did mean that they had to disagree with some central formulations in Freud's theories. Clara Thompson was the most balanced of the theorists of neo-Freudianism, as she could see merits in the approaches of so-called dissidents like Adler and Jung, at the same time she wanted to lay claim to the Freudian heritage. By today, at least when it comes to the psychology of women, Horney's ideas are welcomed within established psychoanalysis; and Sullivan's emphasis on the interpersonal nature of the therapeutic relationship is widely acknowledged. Fromm still remains an outsider, and his ideas continue to appear too shocking to be readily accepted as part of the "mainstream." But Clara Thompson's position has simply evaporated; while there is at least an International Erich Fromm Society established in Germany, the work of Clara Thompson remains in a kind of limbo, a no-man's land reserved for people who have seemingly vanished historically.

In my view, it is one of the tasks of intellectual historians not to let such discontinuities in our understanding of the past continue. Thompson, as well as the rest of the neo-Freudians, deserves to be recognized for how they bravely tried to introduce ideas that were once distinctly unwelcome, and yet by now all-too-often taken for granted.

Our own time has become, at least in America, distinctively positivistic, and the technological advances in psychopharmacology are getting the brunt of attention. But in the long run I hope the more humanistic tradition will reassert itself. Diagnoses on the basis of a mythology about brain functioning may fulfill the needs of insurance companies, but enlightened people should still insist on the relevance of values and beliefs to the practice and theory of psychoanalysis. It is impossible, I believe, to imagine any therapeutic engagement without the presence of a significant ethical dimension. Authoritarianism can flourish as readily within the latest biological psychiatry as it ever did in the context of classical psychoanalysis, which in turn was trying to get away from the abuses of power in end-of-the-nineteenth century psychiatry. Reflecting back on Clara Thompson and the neo-Freudian school can remind us of the earlier efforts to challenge therapeutic authority that are distinctly relevant to our problems today. It should always be possible to inquire into the pros and cons of any therapeutic approach. The richer our understanding of the past the better able we should be to deal in an enlightened way with future choices that get offered to us.

BIBLIOGRAPHY

Burston, Daniel, *The Legacy of Erich Fromm* (Cambridge, Mass.: Harvard University Press, 1991).

Green, Maurice R., editor, *Interpersonal Psychoanalysis: The Selected Papers of Clara M. Thompson,* foreword by Erich Fromm (New York: Basic Books, 1964).

Hornstein, Gale A., *To Redeem One Person Is To Redeem the World: The Life of Frieda Fromm-Reichmann* (New York: The Free Press, 2000).

McLaughlin, Neil G., "How to Become a Forgotten Intellectual: Intellectual Movements and the Rise and Fall of Erich Fromm," *Sociological Forum,* Vol. 13, No. 2 (1998), pp. 215-246.

McLaughlin, Neil G., "Why Do Schools of Thought Fail? Neo-Freudianism as a Case Study in the Sociology of Knowledge," *Journal of the History of the Behavioral Sciences,* Vol. 34, No. 2 (Spring 1998), pp. 113-34.

Ruth Moulton, "The Role of Clara Thompson in the Psychoanalytic Study of Women," in *Women and Analysis: Dialogues on Psychoanalytic Views on Femininity,* ed. Jean Strouse (New York: Grossman, 1974), pp. 278-87.

Mullahy, Patrick, *Oedipus: Myth and Complex, A Review of Psychoanalytic Theory* (New York: Grove Press, 1948)

Helen Swick Perry, *Psychiatrist of America: The Life of Harry Stack Sullivan* (Cambridge, Mass.: Harvard University Press, 1982)

Sue A. Shapiro, "Clara Thompson: Ferenczi's Messenger with Half a Message," in *The Legacy of Sandor Ferenczi,* ed. Lewis Aron and Adrienne Harris (Hillsdale, N.J.: The Analytic Press, 1993), pp.159-73.

PREFACE

IN RECENT YEARS NEW TRENDS AND DEVELOP-
ments in psychoanalysis have emerged. As is usual in scientific progress, the new ideas are not accepted by all workers.
There is a conservative force tending to resist change and a
progressive force pushing forward with impatience. Splits
have occurred and each group tends to isolate itself from the
others. The serious student seeking orientation in the field
finds himself in a state of confusion. On the one hand, many
classical analysts minimize the differences between their point
of view and that of the more culturally oriented groups.
Their thesis is that classical Freudian analysis also recognizes
factors rising out of specific cultural pressures and that the
difference is more one of terminology than ideology. Sullivan, for example, according to them, is saying almost the same
things as Freud, but in different words. On the other hand,
deviant groups have perhaps tended to exaggerate the differences, to imply that Freud is completely outmoded and that
theirs is the only true orientation. The truth has seemed to
me to lie somewhere inbetween. The problem is to obtain
some objectivity in evaluating the picture. Because of the frequent questions asked by students seeking to make a decision
about their own training, I began to review the whole field.

Since psychoanalysis is a theory and method of therapy designed to help the human being master his difficulties in living, the material to be observed and worked with must be the same in every school of psychoanalytic thinking. It must be the human personality especially in its relation to other human personalities. Since the facts are the same, there must be a thread of continuity which runs through the whole picture. Every school, no matter how deviant, must have observed and interpreted some of the same data as every other school. It occurred to me that possibly if one stopped emphasizing differences and tried to note the general stream of development, one would find that this infant science, or (if you prefer) art has a forward moving direction to which all of the different schools have contributed.

Out of this thinking grew a course of lectures which I have been giving for the past several years in the Washington School of Psychiatry in Washington and The William Alanson White Institute of Psychiatry in New York. In response to repeated requests from the students to have these lectures in permanent form I have written this book. I owe much to the students' enthusiasm and probing questions in further developing and clarifying my ideas.

In the course of studying this problem I noted that psychoanalysis developed as probably most sciences do. First there was empirical observation and deductions drawn therefrom. Later, a body of theory began to develop which tended to organize the thinking but at the same time to limit free speculation. Whenever new data could no longer be explained by the theory, or the methods in use were not adequate in new situations, new paths were found and new ideas were introduced. Thus psychoanalysis has developed and changed in sixty years. It has increased its scope—it has been influenced by new discoveries such as those of cultural anthropology and neurophysiology, and it offers a more effective and comprehensive method of therapy today than Freud could have possibly envisioned.

I have tried to be objective in this book but, being human, I must have blind spots. Therefore, I wish to set forth my own psychoanalytic background so that the reader may be able to make allowances for me also. I was first trained by Adolf Meyer, who was always skeptical of the Freudian concepts. However, almost at the same time I came under the influence of psychoanalytic thinking at St. Elizabeth's Hospital, where Edward Kempf and Lucile Dooley, as early as 1920, were applying psychoanalytic methods to the treatment of psychotics. Thus almost from the beginning I had to reconcile two quite different systems of therapy. I found elements in each which supplemented the other. About 1925 I first met Harry Stack Sullivan and became interested in his therapeutic approach to schizophrenia. In 1928 I went to Budapest to study with Ferenczi and found myself in the midst of his experimentation with his "relaxation" therapy. I found Sullivan's and Ferenczi's approach more in keeping with my own way of thinking than the classical Freudian methods. Since then I have also been impressed by the ideas of Erich Fromm. In short my slant is towards the cultural interpersonal school.

Patrick Mullahy's book *Oedipus Myth and Complex* has paved the way for this one. By bringing together in one book the main theories of all the different schools of psychoanalysis, he has furnished a background for critical discussion. Since he has presented the contributions of the various schools so clearly, it seemed to me unnecessary to repeat all the data here. The two should be considered as companion books.

I wish to thank the following publishers for the privilege of quoting passages from their publications:

The Hogarth Press, Ltd., London: quotations from *Collected Papers* by Sigmund Freud;

Alfred A. Knopf, New York: quotations from *Will Therapy and Truth and Reality* by Otto Rank;

Rinehart & Co., New York: quotations from *Escape From Freedom* by Erich Fromm;

William Alanson White Psychiatric Foundation, Washington, D. C.: quotations from *Conceptions of Modern Psychiatry* by Harry Stack Sullivan;

Orgone Institute Press, New York: quotations from *Character Analysis* by Wilhelm Reich.

I wish also to express my appreciation of Mullahy's contribution to this book. He has participated by criticism and often by furnishing information. He has written several passages. Especially his comprehensive knowledge of Jung's and Rank's work has materially added to the substance of the book. Also his critical evaluation of my thinking about Sullivan and Fromm, I believe, has aided in making the picture more accurate and objective.

I wish further to express my indebtedness to Erich Fromm, Nathan Halper, Janet Rioch, Edward Tauber and Elsa Weihl, who have criticized my manuscript from the point of view of content and style.

PSYCHOANALYSIS:

Evolution and Development

chapter one

INTRODUCTORY SURVEY

Psychoanalysis DID NOT SPRING FULL GROWN from the brow of Freud. It has a history. Nor has there been a straight line of development. Since it evolved under the stress of practical exigencies, it shows gaps, regressions, by-paths, as well as progressions. Hence a historical survey of analysis is necessary for a thorough understanding. In this book I shall attempt to trace its growth from its beginning in hypnosis to its present-day condition.

Psychoanalysis is, first of all, a method and technique of therapy for mental and emotional disorder, around which there has evolved a definite body of theory. Until recent years the guiding mind in its evolution was that of its founder, Sigmund Freud, and psychoanalysts still adhere pretty faithfully to many or all of his basic principles. Although there are still people who tenaciously cling to the early theories—which Freud himself had abandoned or at least subordinated to later developments—as if they were final pronouncements, much that is called psychoanalysis today is very different from what Freud talked about in 1893 in his *Studies in Hysteria.* In short, there are certain points at which psychoanalysis became somewhat different. This can be seen more clearly as one looks back on its course of development.

With this in mind, the years since 1885 can be divided into four main periods.

The first period extends from the beginning of Freud's collaboration with Breuer (about 1885) to around 1900. This was a time of great discovery gleaned from clinical observation. Theories of unconscious motivation, repression, resistance, transference, anxiety and etiology of the neuroses were evolved. The latter two only were subject to later drastic revision.

The second period extends from 1900 to somewhere between 1910 and 1920. It dates from the time when the interest first shifted from the theory that neurosis was produced by sexual traumata to the theory that instinctual sexual development was all important in etiology. It covers the development of the first instinct theories, which drew attention to the biological sexual development of the child. It drew to an end in 1910; that is, a new direction of thinking was started by Adler's attack on the sexual theory of neurosis at this time, followed by Jung's repudiation of Freud's orientation three years later. From 1910 to 1920 Freud also was gradually evolving a new theory granting etiological importance to factors other than sex.

The third period, therefore, began in 1910, although the full significance of its changes was not felt by the main psychoanalytic school of thought until about 1920. This was a time of an enlarging field of interest. A theory about the total personality was emerging. Narcissism came under scrutiny and this plus the discovery of the importance of another drive, aggression, laid the ground work for a new theory of instincts which was finally presented by Freud early in the 1920's. One notes that the period from 1910 to about 1925 was chiefly a period of theoretical expansion with little change in the techniques of therapy.

The fourth period began in the middle 1920's and extends to the present. It may be subdivided roughly into two parts, from 1925 to 1934, and from 1934 to the present. The workers in the earlier years concentrated on finding more effective methods of therapy and on trying to enlarge the therapeutic scope of psychoanalysis. There was a shift of emphasis from concern with recall of the past (the removal of the infantile amnesia) to the understanding of the dynamics of the doctor-patient relationship as observed in treatment. This interest did not disappear after 1934; it became embodied in Sullivan's theory of interpersonal relations. Increased study of comparative cultures in the late 1920's eventually contributed significantly to another challenging of Freud's biological theory of neurosis by the so-called cultural school of analysts, whose thinking began to influence psychoanalysis around 1934. The combination of increased knowledge of social processes and pressures and more concern with the inter-personal aspect of the analytic situation is responsible for the characteristic developments of the present era.

The forerunner of psychoanalysis was hypnosis. Freud was a pupil of Charcot and Breuer—both skilled hypnotists. The earliest discoveries of psychoanalysis were made in connection with hypnosis.[1] Even today remnants of the early method survive in the use of the couch and reliance on the authority of the analyst.

With psychoanalysis, a new attitude to mental illness began. All other methods of therapy aimed at relieving the symptom, not at removing the cause. It was recognized that suggestion and hypnosis, by urging the patient to "forget" his trouble, might actually bury the cause more deeply. Freud with his new therapy aimed to lay bare the roots of neurosis.

During most of the first period, 1885 to 1900, there were two workers: Breuer and Freud. In 1880 Breuer had a patient with many hysterical symptoms whom he was treating by hypnosis. The method of therapy at the time was to put the patient under light hypnosis and then suggest that a particular symptom would disappear. In this case there was a different reaction on the part of the patient from the usual one. During her treatment period she began to talk of past events. These proved to be painful experiences of which she apparently had no memory in the waking state. On each occasion she seemed to recall something in some way connected with one of her symptoms. After the recall the associated symptom disappeared. Soon Breuer and Freud concluded that when a specific memory association for each symptom was found, it was as if something were drained off. There seemed to be a kind of catharsis of the residues of past painful experiences.

---

[1] Sigmund Freud, *Collected Papers*, The Hogarth Press, Ltd., London, 1924, Vol. I, p. 289. "The fundamental fact was that the symptoms of hysterical patients are founded upon highly significant, but forgotten, scenes in their past lives (traumas); the therapy founded upon this consisted in causing them to remember and reproduce these scenes in a state of hypnosis (catharsis); and the fragment of theory inferred from this was that these symptoms represented an abnormal form of discharge for quantities of excitation which had not been disposed of otherwise (conversion)."

Freud became associated with Breuer about 1885 and until 1894 he and Breuer worked together. Something then went wrong; Breuer became disgusted and withdrew.[1] From 1894, for many years, Freud worked alone.

In my opinion, this was the period of Freud's greatest creativeness. No theories he later developed can compare with the brilliance of the early discoveries. Much of what he observed then is still an essential part of psychoanalytic thinking. He showed great courage in pursuing ideas which alienated him from his colleagues and his time, such as his theories about sexual etiology, unconscious forces and transference. In observing the operation of unconscious motivations, he found that not only dreams but symptoms and slips of speech represented processes going on outside conscious awareness. The mechanisms of repression (making an experience unconscious) and resistance (the way in which it is kept unconscious) were described at this time. A first relatively simple formulation of transference (a term to be defined in Chapter 5) was also among his early achievements, although the concept was greatly enlarged later. It was during these years that the shift from hypnosis to the psychoanalytic method was made with the aid of a patient's discovery of the effectiveness of free association. Also Freud made a first formulation of the libido theory, a concept which later became the basis of most of the theory of the sexual etiology of the neuroses. The theory was greatly elaborated after 1900, and it is now the aspect of Freud's thinking most vulnerable to

[1] *Collected Papers*, Vol. I, page 293. "When I later began more and more resolutely to put forward the significance of sexuality in the etiology of neurosis, he [Breuer] was the first to show that reaction of distaste and repudiation which was later to become so familiar to me, but which at that time I had not yet learnt to recognize as my inevitable fate."

critical scientific attack. Another questionable notion, presented by him in 1894, was his theory of the origin of anxiety. This he himself modified later (after 1920).

One group of conclusions made before 1900 proved to be premature and based on too little evidence. The frequency of traumatic sexual experiences in the histories which neurotic patients recounted led him to believe he had discovered the specific etiology of hysteria and obsessional neurosis. Hysteria, he believed, was produced when the patient had been the passive victim of sexual aggression in childhood. The obsessional neurosis seemed to appear in those who had a history of having in childhood been active participators in sexual behavior. This seemed to Freud to account for the prominence of the sense of guilt in obsessional neurotics. Certainly the great insincerity which characterized attitudes about the sexual life in the Victorian era made it a universal problem of the time. Viewed in the light of subsequent knowledge, Freud's mistake lay in thinking that sexual traumata and frustration were the chief or only problems producing neurosis, and in assuming also that the Viennese culture of the 1890's in which they took place was a universal manifestation of human nature.

At any rate, later events made Freud revise his whole idea of etiology, and the new data brought about the second period in psychoanalysis.

From 1900 to about 1910 he was occupied with the working out of new theories. The change came about thus. Freud found that in at least some cases sexual traumata allegedly recalled by the patient proved to be phantasies; no sexual seduction at all could be proved. This seemed to point to the psychic trauma's being the creation of the patient. The patient was sick, then, not from a sexual experience which had happened, but from a product of his own imagination about one which had not happened. This was a blow to Freud's early theory, but undaunted he proceeded to examine the new information.

He soon noted the frequency with which patients imagined the same thing—sexual seduction by a parent. Reasoning from his findings on dreams, Freud concluded that this must be the expression of a wish, a wish unacceptable to one's conscious mind, and which therefore has become repressed. The question arose as to why so many people have this wish. From the associations of patients about this he arrived at his formulation of the Oedipus complex, and eventually he developed an elaborate theory of infantile sexuality. He concluded that the sexual development of the child followed definite patterns and that these patterns left effective marks on the child's way of life. As Freud's interest in these matters developed, he became less concerned with the traumatic theory of neurosis and grew more impressed by constitutional factors.

The emphasis on constitution turned attention away from what we would now call the cultural orientation. The idea that traumatic experiences were important was not completely abandoned, but it assumed less importance, and the impression grew on Freud that the patient fell ill primarily because of the strength of his own instinctual drives. This shift of emphasis had certain unfortunate results. It tended to close his mind to the significance of environment and led him to pay too little attention to the role of the emotional problems of parents in contributing to the difficulties of their children. Freud, who was critical of so many false beliefs and practices of his time, seems to have accepted without question the idea that parents always loved their children and that the child's fears and difficulties were chiefly due to his own innate impulses.

However, there were positive aspects to the new emphasis on constitution. It brought attention to the inevitable sexual interests of children, and this had a definite influence on sexual education both in school and in the home. And it led the way in the discovery of the enormous importance of childhood for subsequent personality development.

In the period from 1900 to 1910 a few physicians were becoming interested in Freud's discoveries. Abraham and Ferenczi were among the early pupils. Bleuler and Jung in their observations with psychotics found Freud's theories helpful in explaining hitherto little understood behavior observable in the more severe mental disorders. Still the psychoanalytic method was thought to have but a limited use in therapy. It was believed to be effective only with hysteria, obsessional neurosis and phobias. This belief lasted until after 1920, although before that time a few attempts were made by several, including Ferenczi, Abraham and even Freud, to apply the method to the treatment of perversions and psychosis.

Around 1910 psychoanalytic theory began to show signs of reaching its first dead end. It was becoming increasingly difficult to explain all the data presented by patients within the limited framework of sexual drives. There was a growing realization that to understand the roots of neurosis one must study the total personality.

Prior to this period Freud had thought of man as having two great drives, the sexual drive and the self-preservation drive (ego drive), but he had been of the opinion that the ego drive did not produce neurosis and was incapable of repression.[1] So he had paid no attention to it and the concept was nebulous. The exclusive interest in sexual etiology was first attacked at about this period by two of Freud's pupils, Adler and Jung. Each presented a new theory of neurosis differing greatly from Freud's. Nor did the theory of the one have any essential points in common with that of the other. Their only agreement was rejection of the sexual concept of neurosis.

Adler first seriously differed with Freud in 1910. He saw man's problem as a struggle for power in an attempt to overcome a feeling of inferiority. He was really the first person to point out that nonsexual elements had a role in neurosis and he was the first one to think of neurosis as having to do with the character pattern and the ego drive. In fact one of Freud's criticisms of Adler was that he attempted to explain the whole character of a person instead of limiting his theory to an understanding of illness.

The second pupil to disagree decisively with Freud was Jung, who left the psychoanalytic group in 1913. He too was opposed to the emphasis on sex. He believed man was also influenced by other forces, that there was a higher nature in

[1] This early conception of the ego should not be confused with Freud's later formulation of it in *The Ego and the Id.*

him with which the animal nature had to be reconciled and which played a part in creating conflict. Jung redefined the term libido; he thought of it as a general life energy. He thought that even if it had once had a sexual origin, it was no longer reducible to sexual terms.

Freud could not accept many of the views of Adler and Jung. He found Adler too superficial, and felt that both Adler and Jung discarded that which was most characteristic of analysis. The controversy was bitter and the separation was final. Both men undoubtedly had contributions to make to psychoanalysis and it is unfortunate that they became cut off from the main stream.

At any rate, the questioning of basic psychoanalytic theory started by these two men was an extreme indication of a need for expansion of thinking. Freud first met this with a more precise definition of the relation of libido to narcissism (to be discussed later), and during the years immediately following he finally became interested in examining the ego drives and developing a theory of the total personality.

The war of 1914–18 further focused attention on ego drives. The traumatic neuroses of war again raised the question about sexual etiology. It was found that soldiers who became neurotically ill as a result of war experiences had a type of dream not easily explained by Freud's theory. In their dreams they tended to relive recent traumatic experiences. This, Freud felt, could not be interpreted as sexual wish fulfillment. His interest in these dreams started the development of his concept of the repetition compulsion.

Another idea came into analysis around this period, possibly also stimulated by studying the war neuroses, and that

was that aggression as well as sex might be an important repressed impulse. Adler had already pointed this out, but later
Freud came to it in his own way. The puzzling problem was
how to include it in the theory of instincts. It seemed to be a
function of the self-preservation drive and yet was related to
sex through sadism (sexual pleasure in producing pain).
Eventually Freud solved this by his second instinct theory.
Aggression found its place as part of the death instinct. It is
interesting that normal self-assertion, i.e., the impulse to master, control or come to self-fulfilling terms with the environment, was not especially emphasized by Freud.

We cannot now go into all the new theories presented by
Freud in the early 1920's—Eros and the death instinct, the
repetition compulsion, the new division of personality into
Ego, Superego and Id, a new theory of anxiety. These
changed radically the theoretical structure of psychoanalysis
but had remarkably little effect on its application to patients.
That is, although new theories were developed, no new
methods of therapy appeared except in the Adlerian and
Jungian schools. The successful application of theory to
therapy was still limited to a few types of cases, although as
knowledge of psychoanalysis was spreading people with all
kinds of emotional difficulties were seeking treatment in increasing numbers. By 1920 psychoanalysis as a method of
therapy was at its lowest ebb. Enough years had gone by to
show that psychoanalysis as it was practiced did not bring
permanent cure. It also had become clear that neurosis is a
disease of the total personality and that therapy, to be effective, must take this into consideration.

Freud at this time began to turn from his interest in

therapy to an interest in understanding society. Here, although he wrote several books based on his extensive observations of human nature, he was handicapped by lack of knowledge of comparative cultures and by his bias in favor of a biological theory. He became increasingly pessimistic and his final paper on therapy, "Analysis Terminable and Interminable," [1] brought his biological thinking to its logical dead end.

However, although Freud himself was pessimistic about therapy by the early 1920's, already forces were at work seeking a solution. Rank and Ferenczi were the leaders in the search for new techniques. Both felt that analysis had become too much of an intellectual process, that too much emphasis was placed on recalling the past, and that this often meant that analysis was not a living emotional experience. Wilhelm Reich also made an important contribution in presenting a method of character analysis. Harry Stack Sullivan in America was beginning his researches, which were to demonstrate that some psychotics could be reached by analytic methods.

Out of the various researches emerged a new aim for therapy. The old goal had been the recovery of the infantile amnesia. It had been thought that the bringing of past experiences into consciousness produced the cure. So the patient had been urged always to think about his childhood. The new approach, first advocated by Rank and Ferenczi, was based on the assumption that the patient did not suffer so much from his past as from the way in which his past was influencing his present behavior. This was seen more clearly by Rank than by Ferenczi. This concept is too complicated to

[1] *International Journal of Psychoanalysis,* Vol. XVIII, October, 1937, pp. 373-405.

be explained in an introductory chapter. The important thing for our present purposes is to see that this placing of emphasis on the present drew more attention to the doctor-patient relationship; this shift of emphasis from the past to the present made possible the developments characteristic of the fourth period. Out of observing how the patient was behaving in the analysis came Reich's theory of character defenses, an interest in studying more fully the activities of the ego, and the theory of interpersonal relations.

Ferenczi, Reich and Anna Freud, while making significant contributions to the new interests, still did not question any of the fundamental tenets of Freud's instinct theories. Rank, Horney, Fromm and Sullivan discarded the instinct theories. Rank especially was not satisfied with Freud's negative defensive evaluation of the ego. Later Horney and Fromm each developed theories of the origin of character based on other premises, chiefly cultural and interpersonal. The increased interest in the analytic situation produced a new development, formulated separately by Sullivan, Ferenczi and Rank. This was that the analytic situation is an active relationship between two people, that one cannot eliminate a consideration of the personality of the analyst as playing a part in the process. Jung also had stressed this earlier, but not as clearly and comprehensively.

Beginning about 1933 there were indications of further changes. Horney's book, *The Neurotic Personality of Our Time,* was one of the first definite presentations of a new orientation stressing the importance of cultural and environmental influences in neurosis. It has been said that Freud always took cultural forces into consideration, and it is probable that he did so even more than he himself knew. However, his theoretical approach stressed biology. The new approach discarded the libido theory and presented a new concept of man and his relation to society.

Psychoanalysis has developed in many directions in recent years. The application of the findings of anthropology and sociology to the problems of human behavior is definitely leading away from emphasis on instinct and constitution. We are in a position today to do what Freud could not do, observe the effects of different cultures on the individuals in them. This has shown us that much that Freud believed to be innate biological human nature was to a great extent a reaction to European culture. On the other hand, new interest is developing in the relation of the emotions to somatic disease, and this may eventually throw new light on constitution.

It is not unimportant that analysis in its short life has lived through momentous changes in European culture. Beginning in the Victorian era it has seen the emancipation of women, momentous economic changes, wars, unemployment and depression, and a very great weakening of the power of religion. These changes have produced new problems for man and some of the older ones have become less important. The difficulties attendant on repressed sexuality were a more prevalent preoccupation in the 1890's than they are today.

Modifications in theory and practice have not been accepted uniformly by all analysts. Today there still are those who work almost exclusively with Freud's early ideas, who see neurosis in terms of libido, who believe the Oedipus complex is the central problem. Some even still believe that only hysteria, obsessions and phobias are suitable cases for analysis.

There is, however, a much larger group, especially among American analysts, who have kept Freud's terminology but interpret it very liberally. These people, trained in American psychiatry with its emphasis on the interpersonal aspects of family life, have also been much influenced by the discoveries of cultural anthropology. Their orientation has led them to a more flexible use of Freud's theories, especially in the practical application to therapy. It is a difficult middle course to maintain.

The third group of analysts, of whom the leaders are Horney, Fromm and Sullivan, are more open in their rejection of libido concepts, and have a different view of the nature of man and his relation to society. Their ideas will be discussed extensively in this book.

I shall now consider the development of the fundamental ideas of Freud and subsequent workers in psychoanalysis as these ideas have evolved over the years.

chapter two

EVALUATION OF FREUD'S
BIOLOGICAL ORIENTATION

THE LIBIDO THEORY

THE BEST KNOWN ASPECT OF FREUD'S WORK perhaps and, at the same time, the most controversial is the libido theory. Beginning in the 1890's with a relatively simple concept constructed along lines analogous to electrodynamics or hydrodynamics, Freud eventually created two elaborate instinct theories, in both of which the distribution and function of the libido played an important part. The early formulation reads as follows:

"I should like . . . to dwell for a moment on the hypothesis which I have made use of . . . I mean the conception that among the psychic functions there is something which should be differentiated (an amount of affect, a sum of excitation), something having all the attributes of a quantity—although we possess no means of measuring it—a something which is capable of increase, decrease, displacement and discharge, and which extends itself over the memory-traces of an idea like an electric charge over the surface of the body. We can apply this hypothesis . . . in the same sense as the physicist employs the conception of a fluid electric current." [1]

The concept of libido took its origin from the attempt to explain such phenomena as hysteria. Freud thought that in this disease sexual energy was blocked from its normal outlet and that it then flowed into other organs and became "bound" or contained at various points, manifesting itself in symptoms. He discovered that patients whom he treated had been in good health until "an intolerable idea" presented itself to them. In other words, they were confronted by an experience, a feeling, an idea so painful that they resolved to forget it since they felt unable to resolve the incompatibility between the experience and their ego (as Freud expresses it) by the usual processes of thought, that is, by reason. Freud found that unbearable ideas developed chiefly in connection with sexual experiences and sensations. Patients could clearly recollect their efforts not to think of such experiences, that is, to suppress them. This he thought furnished the necessary background for various pathological reactions, namely hysteria, obsessions, hallucinatory psychoses. The efforts of the ego to treat the unbearable idea as "non arrivée" failed in that the memory-trace and the affect attached to it have made a permanent impression on the psyche. They cannot be extirpated. However, if the ego succeeds in transforming a strong idea into a weak one, that is, depriving it of its affect (the quantity of excitation with which an idea is charged), a kind of solution of the problem confronting the ego [2] is achieved. But the quantity of excitation detached from the idea must be utilized. In the case of hysteria the unbearable

[1] *Collected Papers*, Vol. I, p. 75.
[2] "Ego" here has not yet become clearly defined.

idea was said to be made innocuous by the "transmutation" into some bodily form of expression of this quantity of excitation which had been attached to the idea, a process which was called *conversion*. This conversion may be either partial or total and may "proceed" along motor or sensory paths of innervation.

In regard to obsessions and phobias, the affect detached from its idea attached itself to other ideas not of themselves intolerable. Freud's experience led him to believe that unbearable ideas most frequently arose in regard to the sexual life. The obsession is a surrogate for an unbearable sexual idea, having taken the latter's place in consciousness. "The detachment of the sexual idea from its affect," he says, "and the connection of the latter with another idea, suited to it but not intolerable, are processes which occur outside consciousness—they may be presumed but they cannot be proved by any clinical-psychological analysis . . ." [1]

An example which Freud gives of a patient suffering from obsessions will illustrate concretely how Freud used these ideas in therapy.

"A young woman who in five years of married life had only one child complained to me of an obsessive impulse to throw herself from the window or balcony, and also the fear of stabbing her child which seized her at the sight of a sharp knife. She confessed that marital relations seldom occurred, and only with precautions against conception; but she added that this was no privation to her as she was not of a sensual nature. I ventured to tell her that at the sight of a man she had erotic ideas and that she had therefore lost confidence in

[1] *Collected Papers*, Vol. I, p. 67.

herself and regarded herself as a depraved person, capable of anything. The re-translation of the obsession into the sexual was successful; in tears she confessed at once to her long-concealed misery in her marriage and later on related in addition some painful thoughts of an unchanged sexual nature, such as the often-recurring sensation of something forcing itself under her skirts." [1]

We can see the further development of the concept of libido in what Freud called anxiety-neurosis, of which anxious expectation is said to be the nuclear symptom. This anxious expectation may or may not be conscious, but, if not, it can erupt into consciousness without being evoked by a train of thought, bringing about an anxiety attack.

In anxiety-neurosis, Freud surmised, there is *"a quantum of anxiety in a free floating condition,* which in any state of expectation controls the selection of ideas, and is ever ready to attach itself to any suitable ideational content." [2]

In some cases of anxiety-neurosis no etiology was recognizable. Here evidence "of a grave hereditary taint" was said to be as a rule not difficult to establish. When there was reason to regard such a neurosis as acquired, "careful enquiry to that end reveals a series of injurious conditions (*noxiae*) and influences within the sexual life as important factors in the etiology." [3] Freud is very unclear about these sexual "noxiae"; they have to do with unsatisfactory sexual relations.[4] Thus *coitus interruptus* is mentioned as creating a sexual noxia. Freud thought that such a practice disturbed

---

1 *Collected Papers,* Vol. I, p. 71.
2 *Collected Papers,* Vol. I, p. 80.
3 *Collected Papers,* Vol. I, p. 87.
4 Compare *Collected Papers,* Vol. I, pp. 281-283.

spontaneous sexual discharge sufficiently to produce a cumulative effect which would dispose one to anxiety-neurosis, or, along with other conditions, eventuate in anxiety-neurosis. It was presumed to arise from insufficient sexual satisfaction, which resulted in accumulated somatic excitation of a sexual nature. Freud also observed that in many cases there was a very noticeable abatement of "sexual libido" (conscious sexual feeling) or "psychical desire." [1] The somatic sexual excitation was not assimilated psychically, as Freud expressed it, and was deflected subcortically. In sexual abstinence, for example, the specific activity which follows on "libido," on conscious sexual feeling, was foregone. Two consequences might ensue: accumulation of somatic excitation and then dissipation "along other paths" than along the "path to the mind." Libido then would subside and the excitation would express itself subcortically as anxiety.

In attempting to explain anxiety-neurosis, Freud puts forth the following view of the sexual process as it relates to men, though in essential respects, he says, it applies to women also: "In the sexually mature male organism somatic sexual excitation is produced—probably continuously—and periodically acts as a psychical stimulus. In order to define this idea more clearly, let us interpolate that this somatic sexual excitation takes the form of pressure on the walls of the *vesiculae seminales,* which are lined with nerve-endings; this visceral excitation will then actually develop continuously, but only when it reaches a certain height will it be sufficient to over-come the resistance in the paths of conduction to the cerebral cortex and express itself as a psychical stimulus. Thereupon

[1] The term libido here is not used in its later technical sense.

the constellation of sexual ideas existing in the mind becomes charged with energy and a psychical state of libidinous tension comes into existence, bringing with it the impulse to relieve this tension. The necessary psychical relief can only be effected by what I shall describe as a *specific* or *adequate activity*. For the male sexual impulse this adequate activity consists in a complicated spinal reflex act resulting in the relief of the tension at these nerve-endings and in all the preparatory psychical processes necessary to induce this reflex. Nothing but the adequate activity would be effective; for, once it has reached the required level, the somatic sexual excitation is continuously transmuted into psychical excitation; the activity which will free the nerve-endings from burdensome pressure and so abolish the whole of the somatic excitation present, thus allowing the subcortical tracts to reestablish their resistance, must absolutely be carried into operation." [1]

When somatic sexual excitation, for some reason, cannot be assimilated psychically, the excitation is often not dissipated by appropriate activity and is expended subcortically in anxiety. Thus the symptoms of anxiety-neurosis are said to be in some measure surrogates for the specific activity normally following sexual excitation.

It is instructive to study Freud's comparison of hysteria with anxiety-neurosis. He claimed that the latter is the somatic counterpart of the former. He says that in each there is (1) an accumulation of excitation, (2) a psychical inadequacy resulting in abnormal somatic processes, and (3) a deflection of excitation somatically instead of psychical assim-

[1] *Collected Papers*, Vol. I, pp. 97-98.

ilation. The difference was said to be that in anxiety-neurosis the excitation is purely somatic, while in hysteria it is "purely psychical."

There is another point which is important for understanding Freud's conception of neurosis. He believed that whether a neurotic illness occurs at all depends upon a quantitative factor, on the "total load" of sexual excitation the nervous system could master without, for example, its being discharged in the form of anxiety. There are, however, he said, other conditions such as fright or physical exhaustion through illness which diminish the tolerance of the nervous system.

One can sum up what has been said by the conclusion that neuroses like hysteria, obsessional neurosis, neurasthenia, and anxiety-neurosis have an immediate cause in a special "disturbance of the nervous economy" and that they all have a common source in a disturbance of the sexual life. In neurasthenia and anxiety-neurosis the present sexual life only is concerned. In the other neuroses traumatic events in the past life furnish the disturbance.

Freud's explanation of hysteria is especially enlightening for anyone attempting to understand the evolution of psychoanalytic theory. The specific etiology of hysteria, he believed in the early years, was a passive sexual experience before puberty. As is well known, Breuer and Freud, in investigating hysteria, discovered that a patient under hypnosis revealed certain things of which he was unaware in his normal waking state. Under hypnosis recollections were aroused by interrogating the patient which revealed the events which occurred to produce the symptom. Freud in using "the probing procedure of J. Breuer" traced hysterical symptoms to their origin, invariably an experience in the person's sexual life. The specific cause of hysteria was said to be an event or the memory of an event connected with the person's sexual life, having two very important features. "The event, the unconscious image of which the patient has retained, is a premature sexual experience with actual stimulation of the genitalia, the result of sexual abuse practised by another person, and the period of life in which this fateful event occurs is early childhood, up to the age of eight to ten, before the child has attained sexual maturity." [1]

A mental impression of the assault or seduction was said to be retained. At puberty, when the sexual drive is stronger, this unconscious mental impression, under certain conditions, is re-activated. Because of the increased capacity for sexual feeling the repressed memory acquires new force. It now produces the same result as an actual event in the present, an effect which the original experience itself lacked. Such a memory is not conscious. When at puberty it is reawakened, there is a liberation of affect although the ideas associated with it remain repressed. Unconscious memories of this kind are said to have an associative and logical connection with ideas which are not acceptable to the person's moral values and beliefs. Hence, the ego represses all such ideas.

Symptoms of hysteria occur only when the memories of childhood sexual experiences are unconscious; if they have always been conscious, according to Freud, hysteria does not result.

It was not long before Freud made a very bewildering

[1] *Collected Papers*, Vol. I, pp. 148-149.

discovery: the stories of childhood seduction and assault which patients related often were phantasies, not accounts of actual occurrences, being attempts at defense "against the memory of sexual activities by the child himself." [1]

Freud then made a fateful revision of theory. Hitherto he had thought that, in the main, accidental experiences in childhood produced a specific predisposition to hysteria and obsessional neurosis. Now he concluded that heredity and constitution must be the important etiological factors in the psycho-neuroses. Sexual constitution now began to occupy his attention more and more. In other words, the nature of the psycho-neurosis was now thought to lie in disturbances of the sexual processes, "of those organic processes which determine the development and form of expression of the sexual craving." [2] And so whatever has a harmful effect on the sexual processes belongs to the etiology of the neuroses. This early formulation of the role of sexuality in the neuroses remained essentially unchanged in Freud's thinking until he modified it somewhat in the second instinct theory.

Whatever one may think of Freud's theoretical orientation, he made the enormously significant discovery that childhood experiences are of the greatest importance for subsequent personality development; and that the effects of such experiences continue to operate outside conscious awareness. It happened that his first discoveries were made in connection with hysteria, where strong early sexual interests accompanied by strong prohibitions against them are frequently discovered as originating factors. Hysteria is seen much less

[1] *Collected Papers*, Vol. I, p. 276.
[2] *Collected Papers*, Vol. I, p. 282.

frequently today; it seems possible that cultural changes account to some extent for its disappearance, and that it is more prominent whenever the sexual life is hedged in as it was in the Victorian era. At any rate, the frequency of hysteria in his patients during the years when Freud was first formulating his theories may well have been the decisive influence in bringing to his attention the significance of repressed sexuality in neurosis.

Freud's turning away from environmental factors, as a major concern, to organic constitution was, however, most unfortunate. For this reason, he came to minimize what actually happens between people, failed to take into consideration what more recent observation suggests, that it is the dynamic interaction between people which provides the locus of functional mental illness. He fell back upon organic constitution in order to find an explanatory principle for organizing and interpreting observed facts. Because of his experiences, he limited his attention, at least for a long time, largely to those aspects of organic processes which have to do with sex.

THE FIRST INSTINCT THEORY

The discovery, around 1900, that some of the early childhood traumatic experiences described by patients were phantasies had a far reaching effect on the development of psychoanalytic theory. Although, regrettably, it turned Freud's interest away from studying the interaction of people, it opened up a new and important field, the early development of the child. In spite of the fact that Freud concentrated his interest almost exclusively on the sexual aspects of this development, nevertheless his work constitutes one of the first studies in child development, and the observations made had a revolutionary effect on educational attitudes towards children. Freud first became interested in trying to discover why patients so frequently made up phantasies of early sexual seduction, and it was in the search for understanding of this that he developed a theory of the sexual development of man.

The theory that libido (sexual energy) was the vital force in neurosis had already been propounded by him. This he included in his instinct theory as one of the two great drives in life. These were, then, a drive for self-preservation and a drive for procreation (the preservation of the species). His first instinct theory was based on the idea that these two forces dominated human behavior. The self-preservation instinct, he believed, created no neurotic problem. Its needs could not be denied for any length of time without serious danger to life. Therefore, its energy could not accumulate as could the sexual energy or libido, as already described. Consequently, for many years, although Freud's first instinct theory assumed that life was dominated by a pair of instincts, he paid no attention to the possible influence of the self-preservation instinct and devoted all of his energies to working out possible paths followed by the sexual instinct, that is, the vicissitudes of the libido.

He soon discovered the importance of a set of reactions to which he gave the name Oedipus complex, taking the name from the Greek myth of Oedipus, who slew his father and married his mother, crimes which brought dire consequences and for which he atoned by blinding himself. The complex as described by Freud contains a comparable situation. He observed, primarily from the recollections of neurotics and from dream interpretation, that a child at a certain age regularly becomes sexually interested in the parent of the opposite sex and develops a feeling of rivalry and a wish to displace the parent of the same sex. Freud concluded that this was a universal phenomenon occurring between three and five years of age, and for some time he believed all neurosis took its origin in this situation, that in fact neurosis could not originate in experiences occurring at an earlier time. The problematical aspect of the Oedipus complex was thought to be due to the following. The boy child, for example, soon learns that sexual interest in the mother is tabu. Also, because of his erotic interest in his mother he feels hostile to his father, whom he considers a rival. But he loves his father at the same time, and this makes hostile feelings towards him a source of distress. Also, because of his hostile feelings toward his father and his sexual feelings for his mother he expects punishment, and the punishment which fits the crime is castration. Something similar happens to the little girl with the father as the center of erotic interest, but in her case the fear of castration plays little part in the conflict because she has no penis to lose. This early sexual interest in the parents, Freud believed, was the source of the adult neurotic's phantasies of seduction in childhood. The phantasies were the expression of a wish to have their "Oedipus" interests gratified without guilt.

Presently Freud found there was more to the story of neurosis than the Oedipus complex. There was increasing evidence that some conditions began at an even earlier age. This led to a study of what Freud called the pregenital stages of the libido. At this point in his theory the word "sexual" was given a new meaning in psychoanalysis. Prior to this time when Freud talked of sex he meant sex, that is, erotic feelings connected with the genital organs. From this point on the term sexual came to be applied to any pleasurable body sensation, and in addition through the notion of sublimation it was applied to emotions not strongly identified with any one part of the body, such as tenderness and affection and even such feelings as satisfaction in work. This is very confusing and has led to much misunderstanding of Freud. He wished to emphasize by this that the energy concerned in all these activities was libido, which he considered to be sexual in origin.

Much later (1914), in his paper on Narcissism,[1] he hypothecated an erotic component attached to all organs of the body generated by the organs themselves. This idea further extended the psychoanalytic meaning of the word "sexual."

He suggested that three orifices of the body, the mouth, anus and genitals, were especially endowed with libido, and he noted that there seemed to be a uniform order of development of interest and satisfaction in these three parts. The first organ of interest for the child is the mouth. For the newborn infant this is the all-absorbing organ of pleasure. Through it he makes contact with the first object of libido, the mother's breast. In the absence of the breast he hallucinates contact with it by sucking his thumb. Freud likened the infant's bliss after nursing to the relaxation after orgasm.[2] This was seen as the first pregenital stage of development. Abraham later divided this stage into two parts, the earlier

[1] *Collected Papers*, Vol. IV, Ch. 3.
[2] Sigmund Freud, *Three Contributions to the Theory of Sex*, Nervous and Mental Disease Publishing Company, New York, 1930, p. 43.

characterized by sucking pleasure and the later by biting pleasure.

According to Freud, towards the end of the first year of life the center of libidinal interest begins to shift to the anal region, and the infant's chief source of erotic pleasure becomes connected with retention and expulsion of feces. This, he noted also, is related to the parents in terms of defiance and submission and has much to do with a developing feeling of power. The child discovers that the retention and expulsion of feces excites great interest in those who care for him. By prolonged withholding he can reduce the parent at times to distraction, or by choosing his own ways of expulsion he can arouse feelings of annoyance and exasperation in those responsible for his care, and he presently learns that submitting to the parent's wishes gains approbation. The tendency to have an active or passive attitude towards life first becomes apparent at this time. It is evident that in describing this stage Freud is, in fact if not in intention, describing much more than the possible erotic pleasures connected with the anal zone. He is describing also a complex interpersonal situation.

The next place the libido has as its object of interest is the penis, ushering in the phallic stage, which is the third pregenital stage of libidinal development. At about the age of three the penis becomes the center of erotic pleasure for both sexes—the clitoris being the substitute in the female. Freud believed that the little girl at this time is unaware of her vagina and that she believes she too must count on her clitoris-"penis" for pleasure. This "phallic" stage of libido development is the period at which penis envy develops in little girls. The sexual interest in the penis at first is not related to an external object; that is, it is auto-erotic; but presently this stage merges into that of sexual interest in the parents, and genital excitations presumably become associated with Oedipus wishes already described. The Oedipus period, Freud believed, comes to an end for two reasons: the child temporarily loses interest in his organ because due to the fact that it has not yet matured he cannot understand its full significance. The threat of castration and fear of his own death wishes against his father because of the desire for exclusive possession of his mother also make the boy turn away from the Oedipus situation. The girl, because she has no penis to lose, is more likely to prolong the Oedipus phase.

Out of the two facts, lack of knowledge and castration threat, comes the latency period, during which sexual interests are allegedly dormant or at least greatly reduced. This extends to pre-puberty, when increased functioning of the sex glands leads to re-awakening of sex interests.

Increased production of libido at puberty makes for restlessness, and a search for an object ensues. Usually there is a revival of erotic interest in the parents for a short period, but unless a serious fixation exists, the adolescent soon turns his sexual interests towards more suitable objects. Freud thought the turning away from the parents at this point was aided by the incest tabu.

At puberty the two sexes take different paths of development. The boy maintains his penis interest and so continues along the same lines as in his earlier growth. But for the girl there is a change of direction because, so Freud believed, up to this time she has been unaware of her vagina as a pleasure organ. Her sole interest has been in her clitoris and her desire to be boyish. At puberty she must become aware of her feminine function, renounce the clitoris and accept the passive role. If she had strong penis envy or strong constitutional masculine trends, this is difficult for her and she develops resentment at being a woman.

It is important to remember that Freud presented this as an innate instinctual development. He believed that the libido progressed along the paths we have just outlined and that this was the normal biological sequence of human nature.

His theories of fixation and regression are formulated on the basis of this hypothesis. Fixation occurs when for traumatic or constitutional reasons there is especially strong emphasis on some phase in the course of development resulting in an especially strong binding of the libido at that point. Some portions of the libido never advance beyond this phase. Freud leaned more and more towards emphasizing the constitutional factor. When a fixation exists, if at any point a certain degree of frustration occurs in the forward movement of the libido, it tends to flow back over the previous stages and come to rest at the point of fixation. This flowing back is called regression. Thus in the hysteric there is allegedly a regression of the libido to the phallic stage, and in the obsessional to the anal stage.

In developing the first instinct theory, while postulating two drives as controlling human life (the self-preservation drive and the sex drive) Freud, as I have shown, concentrated his interests almost exclusively on the course of the sexual drive. He was convinced that it and it only was concerned in producing neurosis.

However, he later modified his thinking and concluded that another important drive could also contribute to neurotic difficulties. This resulted in the formulation of the second instinct theory. Since the second theory for the most part adds to rather than modifies the first, it is important to evaluate the first one at this point. There is much genuine observation in it but also much untenable theory. I shall attempt to distinguish between the two.

Freud's errors in theory were of two general types. He often mistook cultural phenomena for biological-instinctual phenomena. Some of the stages of development are definitely products of this culture. Even when it is pretty clear that there are strong biological elements, these are not always sexual in nature. Freud placed all the emphasis on the erotization of a situation when it may have been purely developmental; that is, a stage in the process of growing appearing when the nerve paths are adequately developed. For instance, to be consistent with Freud's theory, a child learns to stand upright and learns to take his first steps because of the erotic pleasure from such use of his muscles. It seems much more likely that it happens because nerve pathways and muscles are sufficiently developed for the next stage in growth. That erotic satisfaction sometimes accompanies these steps may be true but, if so, it is probably usually a subsidiary or incidental fact.[1]

[1] According to Adler the satisfaction experienced would be due to the feeling of power. According to Sullivan the achievement would produce a genuine non-neurotic feeling of power.

When we consider the stages in Freud's scheme in the light of these criticisms, it will be found that the general order of development in our society has been accurately observed by him and that the stages may be re-evaluated in the light of other data. The oral stage seems to be chiefly determined by biological development. The newborn infant is chiefly a mouth. The most developed part of the cortex at birth is that which governs the oral zone. We are justified in assuming that the infant contacts the world and comprehends it in the beginning primarily in terms of mouth. We, however, question whether the erotic satisfaction obtained is the determining factor. It seems more likely that he contacts the world by mouth because it is his most adequate organ. Thus the oral stage is organically determined but not primarily because of its pleasure value.

Moreover, the kind of world contacted through the mouth is not universally the same, and the differences in experience make a more significant impression on personality development than does the organic fact of a period of oral primacy. There occur in different cultures variations as to the length of time a child is customarily breast fed and also variations in frequency of feeding. In some a child may nurse over a period of many years in contrast to our own system where the tendency has been to shorten the period of nursing as much as possible. Also among many peoples the child is fed whenever he cries, while with us until very recently a rigid schedule was not only enforced but considered good for the child. Moloney, in his study of the Okinawans, maintains that the free nursing habits of these people are the basis of their flexible, loving, anxiety-free personalities.[1] Thus although there is an organic base for the oral stage, its effect on the personality of the child is undoubtedly greatly influenced by the cultural attitude towards it.

When we come to what Freud calls the anal stage, cultural factors dominate the picture. In organic terms there occurs a time when the child can easily master his anal sphincter. This time is later than the period of oral mastery, but except for this general consideration the exact time of appearance is not determined organically but by cultural influences. The child's interest allegedly becomes focused on the pleasure of defecation and retention of feces. However, it is clear from Freud's description that much more than animal pleasure in feces is involved. What Freud describes chiefly is the child's reactions to toilet training. He assumes that these follow of necessity. Today it is known that in different cultures there are great variations in methods of toilet training; also in some it occurs earlier than in others and in some it seems to be not at all important. Consequently, Freud's description applies especially to this culture.

The emphasis at this stage belongs not on the pleasure the child gets from retaining and expelling feces, but on the struggle with the parents. The child's wish to do what he wants whenever he wishes comes here for the first time into sharp conflict with the parents' plans. This is what puts its stamp on the character of the child. Parents who set a great

[1] James Clark Moloney, *The Magic Cloak*, Montrose Press, Wakefield, Mass., 1949, pp. 302-303. I do not agree with Moloney that the nursing situation is the primary causal factor in moulding character, but the nursing situation itself is a result of and at the same time an expression of the complicated network of a particular cultural pattern.

store on regularity and neatness usually have in their whole attitude to life rigidities and rituals which are also forced on the child. (In fact these pressures have their effect even earlier than the anal stage.) What pleasure the child eventually discovers in controlling his feces may be considered a kind of consolation for his compromise with the parents, who are culture carriers, and not the cause of the biological stage of development.

Parents show a distinct but ambivalent interest in the child's feces. Defecation is a daily event for which he is praised. On the other hand, feces are regarded as dirty if he touches them, and he is a bad boy. Certainly the parents' concern about the control of the evacuation and their interest in the product itself must help to fix the time of the anal stage and contribute markedly to its characteristic nature.

Another point to be questioned here is whether the anal stage of interest necessarily precedes the phallic. The maturing of the nerve pathways of both anus and penis, in so far as they serve as organs of excretion, occurs at about the same time. It is by no means certain that a child would be interested first in his anus and secondly in his phallus if outside forces did not emphasize the anus. It is quite possible that in another culture the child's order of interest might be different.

The phallic phase also has some organic basis. The child does not concern himself specifically with his penis until he is capable of having some control of it. When this time has arrived, children become much absorbed in trying to find out what the penis can do and why boys are different from girls. The pleasurable sensations which can be produced by manipulating the genitals are one of the discoveries. Here both sexes presumably have equal satisfaction from their auto-erotic activities, but there is a marked inequality in the sense of achievement of the two sexes regarding another function of the sexual organ. What the girl seems to envy in the boy is what he can do with his penis, the fact that for example he can direct his urinary stream and shoot it further than she can. This is an organic inequality measured by the standards of childhood and may well be used later as a symbol for other feelings of inequality.

The attitude of the parents also has an important influence on the phallic phase. The child's discovery of the pleasure-producing quality of his genital is often cause for concern to parents in our society. In this particular field of research even today the child in our culture frequently encounters strong disapproval. Where the parents aided him in mastering the uses of the anal sphincter, they frown upon his exploring the erotic functions of the genitals, and out of this cultural atti-tude comes the fear of castration which Freud considered one of the chief sources of anxiety in man. He believed the fear of castration was greatly reinforced by the discovery in this phase of development that little girls lacked penises. This is probably a true observation of little boys who have been scolded for their "naughty" interests. It is by no means cer-tain, however, that a child who has not been obstructed feels threatened at finding that someone else is different from him. To him unprejudiced investigation of sexual differences is conceivably merely another interesting discovery.

Anthropological research has clearly shown now that the Oedipus complex as it is described by Freud is not universal but is a product of monogamous patriarchal society.[1] It develops in situations where a small family group constitutes the child's first interpersonal world. It seems to include much more than erotic reactions. In fact, when the child shows more than a passing interest in the erotic relations with the parents one must seek its source in erotic attitudes of the parent toward the child. In our western culture where families are small and the parent has the chief care of the child, the relation to the parents constitutes the child's first experience in living with his fellow man. Here rivalries, jealousies and hostilities about all sorts of things first come to life. We would question whether sex as such is the invariable cause of the rivalry and hostility. The child plays the parents off against each other as a method of dividing and ruling, as well as feeling hostile to them whenever they obstruct the development of his interests. Only when the parent has an erotic interest in the child is the child's sexual interest stimulated to a point of becoming a problem. It is true, however, that since one of the interests of this period of life is an attempt to understand the possible uses of the genitals, in the course of this investigation the child usually discovers that bodily contact with someone else is somehow connected with it, and this discovery is often made in connection with physical contact with his parents. The eventual effect of this on the child's further development depends on how the parents feel about the situation. If some of their own frustrated erotism finds guilty satisfaction in the child's caresses, the classical

[1] See, for example, *Three Essays on Sex and Marriage* by Edward Westermarck, Macmillan and Company, New York, 1934; and *Sex and Repression in Savage Society* by Bronislaw Malinowski, Harcourt, Brace and Company, New York, 1927.

picture of Freud's Oedipus complex may appear. But this is not universal even in our culture.

The study of comparative cultures has also shown that the latency period, as far as it is real, is a product of our civilization.[1] It probably appears not only because the child's sexual interests are disapproved and repressed but because at this period the world becomes much larger. He goes to school, and the process of becoming part of a group of contemporaries absorbs his interest. I said, as far as it is real. There is a question whether the child's interest in his sexual organs dies out during the so-called latency period even in our society. With an expanded relationship to his playmates and awareness of the disapproval of parents, the child tends to share his interests and experiences with those of his own age and to keep his ideas to himself where his parents are concerned. This situation, I think, is very frequently the fact about the alleged latency period.

The biological facts of puberty are certainly real, and the time of their appearance is fixed by organic development. Also organically a need for erotic satisfaction is very strong. No one can deny the libidinous importance of puberty. Nevertheless, much that Freud observed, especially about girls at this period, can be explained as a reaction to the cultural situation. He assumed that girls know nothing about the vagina until puberty when they discover its meaning and must renounce interest in the clitoris in its favor, and that it is this momentous biological change which produces the specific difficulties in a girl's accepting her femininity. The assumption of ignorance of the vagina prior to puberty is not

---

[1] See Bronislaw Malinowski, *Sex and Repression in Savage Society.*

borne out by clinical facts. Many girls know of it earlier, and discover auto-erotic pleasure in its manipulation. Nor does the girl ever renounce her interest in the clitoris. It remains one of her natural sexual satisfactions throughout life. The resentment that the girl feels at puberty at accepting her femininity does not grow out of the loss of her childhood pleasure organ, but is a reaction to the changed attitude of her environment towards her. She suddenly finds herself hedged in, chaperoned, taught new standards of behavior for herself, and the new rules tend to limit her former free activities. This was even more strongly the case at the time when Freud first described the feminine role. This (the cultural requirement) is the difficult adjustment which girls must master at puberty. Moreover, both sexes must adapt themselves to the fact that in our society the exercise of the newly developed function usually must be postponed for many years. All other capacities can be utilized as soon as they develop. Only here can one genuinely say that a problem is created by the damming of the "libido".

So Freud's theory of instinctual development is important because he observed the general progress of child development in this culture. His conclusion, however, that the driving force was the pursuit of erotic bodily satisfaction is open to question, as is also the idea that all stages are biologically determined.

Specifically we question the idea that the erotic satisfaction of nursing led the infant to concentrate on the mouth zone, that erotic satisfaction of defecation produces the anal stage, etc.

In short because Freud started with the idea that neurosis is produced by damming sexual energy, resulting in a displacement of this energy to various parts of the body, he was led to give pleasure in body sensations a false significance in personality development.

One can understand the biological development of the child better if one discards the concept of libido altogether. One then sees the different stages in terms of growth and of human relations. In the earliest stage the child relates to his environment by his mouth. In the second and third stages he has difficulties with his fellow men over his attitude towards his anus and phallus, etc. Eventually he becomes sufficiently aware of the tabus and restrictions of the culture to conclude it is better to keep many of his body interests to himself. And finally his problem is to find a place for his full-blown sexual drive in the type of life required by the society in which he lives.

Freud's positive contribution is that he observed that the unspoiled child takes great pleasure and interest in his body and all its functions. This was a revolutionary admission in 1900. In the process of mastering the body functions the child may learn to exploit the pleasure aspects, especially if he is unhappy in his human relations. But to say that this latter statement is really what Freud meant is untrue and would confuse the picture. Rather this is a summary of what we have learned as a result of Freud's observations, which called our attention to the processes of child development.

Freud claimed that libidinal pleasure in body functions was important in the dynamics of neurosis, whereas many think today the dynamics of neurosis are derived from other sources. Freud did not envision people in terms of developing powers and as total personalities. He thought of them much more mechanistically—as victims of the search for the release of tension.

Freud presented the libido theory as a scientific hypothesis of the dynamics of human behavior. For this purpose it must fulfill certain requirements. A valid hypothesis must not only give a possible explanation of all the phenomena observed; it should further not hinder investigation. Freud eventually realized that his libido hypothesis could not explain all the phenomena. It failed as a satisfactory explanation of aggression. It also led to untenable conclusions about perversions and narcissism.

According to Freud's theory, "neurosis is the negative of a perversion." [1] That is, neurotic symptoms represent repression of perverse sexual interests. Perversion, on the other hand, does not spring from repression. In the perversions infantile sexual interests remain conscious and receive gratification. Because there is satisfactory discharge of the libido there is no damming of energy and repression does not take place. This logically brought Freud to the conclusion that in the case of perversion there is no neurosis and nothing can be analyzed.

This point of view led to the assumption that overt sexual problems such as homosexuality cannot be analyzed since, according to Freud, in the case of adults all sexual activities except the union of male and female genitals are termed perverse unless they serve as mere forepleasure. Such an attitude towards homosexuality still persists among classical analysts,

[1] *Three Contributions to the Theory of Sex*, p. 28.

although since 1911 when Ferenczi first questioned this premise there have always been a few analysts who were not satisfied
with this formulation. Ferenczi in 1911 reported from his
observations that in at least one type of male homosexual the
homosexuality seemed to be a symptom of neurosis.[1] Freud
expressed dissatisfaction with Ferenczi's calling these homosexuals compulsion-neurotics.[2] However, since in recent years
there have been a few successful analyses of homosexuals, we
have to question Freud's opposing premise, that a perversion
because it discharges its libido is therefore unanalyzable. In
the same way Freud found difficulty in explaining compulsive
heterosexuality or heterosexual promiscuity as neurosis. In
these conditions also since libido is discharged there should
be no repression, according to theory.

    Another point where rigid adherence to the libido formula
led him astray was in the concept of narcissism. Here his
theory also placed narcissism outside the possibility of analysis. In order to fit narcissism into the framework of energy
drives, a very complicated system had to be evolved to explain it. Freud early in his work noted that some people do
not form attachments to others. These people seemed inaccessible to therapy. They developed no relationship to the
physician; that is, they formed no transference.[3] To these people he gave the name of narcissists, taking the name from the
myth of Narcissus. Freud believed that these people were
completely absorbed in loving themselves. This idea seemed
to fit very well into the libido picture. If a quantum of

[1] Sandor Ferenczi, *Sex in Psychoanalysis*, Richard G. Badger, Boston, 1916,
Ch. XII.
[2] Sigmund Freud, *Three Contributions to the Theory of Sex*, p. 11, footnote.
[3] See Chapter 5.

energy did not go out from a person and become attached to another, it seemed logical to suppose it remained attached to the person's own ego.

Freud assumed that originally a quantum of sexual energy was attached to every organ in the body. Such, he said, is the condition of the organism at birth. This is primary narcissism. However, he thought there was no way of measuring this energy except as we presumably can observe it going out and becoming attached to another organism. In doing this the narcissistic libido becomes converted into object libido and a bond is formed between the two people. This is object love.

It is important to keep in mind that Freud thought of this libido as a quantity. If a part of one's libido becomes attached to another person, then the individual has lost it. Freud says that is why a man in love suffers from feelings of unworthiness.[1] He has lost some of his self-love. His ego is poorer in libido. If his love is successful, he gets a quantity of libido back from the other and self-esteem is restored. If a person is rebuffed or falls out of love, his libido then returns to himself and becomes once more attached to his own body. This is secondary narcissism—the return of one's libido to oneself after rebuff. One is again rich in self-love. Primary narcissism Freud saw as healthy; secondary narcissism is always the result of failure to make an object attachment. This is a perfectly consistent theory given the premise that life is dominated by the distribution of libido. However, it puts one in the untenable position of saying that the narcissist is a richer person than the individual capable of love.

[1] *Collected Papers*, Vol. IV, Ch. 3.

As Fromm has pointed out, the facts seem otherwise.[1] Far from being exhausted by loving others one becomes enriched. Also a person capable of genuinely loving himself is by that very fact more capable of loving others. And if he can love one person, he feels more warmth towards many people and his own life is richer. The person incapable of love for others, on the other hand, is in actual fact incapable of loving himself also. All his meticulous attention to his body, his conceit, his general self-centeredness are not evidences of love of self but are attempts to hide the feeling of failure and unlovability. The libido theory, therefore, makes the whole concept of narcissism confusing. It leaves no room for the possibility of seeing that primary and secondary narcissism are totally different kinds of experience. In general in primary narcissism Freud is talking about self-esteem, while secondary narcissism is a defensive device against awareness of loss of self-esteem. Fromm also points out that Freud's theory was consistent with the Protestant cultural standard of the time. The teachings of Luther and Calvin emphasize salvation only through the loss of self and belittling of self. Any concern for the self was considered selfishness and was incompatible with love for others. It is possible that this prevalent cultural attitude kept Freud from seeing that narcissism as clinically observed is not self-love but self-hate.

SECOND INSTINCT THEORY

The third way in which the libido theory proved inadequate was in explaining aggression. It was not until the

[1] Erich Fromm, *Man for Himself*, Rinehart & Co., New York, 1947, pp. 126-141.

period of World War I that Freud turned his attention to the importance of repressed aggression in neurosis. Sadism had been recognized much earlier and had been considered a part of the anal libido. Freud had observed that in the anal stage children first showed tendencies to cruelty and he assumed that this was a part of their constitutional development.[1] He thought that masochism was a secondary development, i.e., it was sadism turned against oneself. He believed that out of the anal stage some quantity of sadistic libido fused with the masculine sexual drive, while a masochistic component became attached to the female sexual drive. Both drives were libidinous in origin. For many years this had seemed to be a satisfactory explanation.

As already indicated, World War I and the neuroses developing in its soldiers had a great deal to do with bringing to Freud's attention the importance of the other instinct he had postulated—the self-preservation instinct. It seemed to him that the neuroses of war were more largely derived from this drive than from sex. This now suggested the problem that perhaps some ego (self-preservation) drives were also important in neurosis and capable of repression.

Aggression seemed not only to be a product of the libido as Freud had postulated in the case of sadism, but there seemed considerable evidence that the self-preservation drive also could produce aggression, and this appeared especially clearly in war. These forces, Freud saw, had also been repressed in our culture, so he could no longer believe that only sexual drives were capable of repression. For several

[1] Subsequently, however, Abraham observed that children showed sadistic tendencies during the later oral stage, and so an oral sadism was found to be prior to the anal stage.

years during and immediately after World War I, Freud seems to have pondered the problem until he finally worked out a reconciliation of the two ideas about aggression.

On the one hand was the old idea of sadism, a part of the sexual drive. On the other hand was aggression, which Freud now saw as destructiveness, and which he believed was not produced by the libido at all.

Another phenomenon came to Freud's attention at about the same time. It seemed that "shell-shocked" soldiers had a different type of dream from that which had been psychoanalytically studied heretofore. In their dreams they tended always to re-live the traumatic situation. Freud questioned that these distinctly unpleasurable dreams could be sexual wish fulfillments; this brought for the first time a doubt of his fundamental theory that the dominating aim of human life was to obtain pleasure, especially sexual satisfaction. Freud now (1918–1922) made the very important discovery that there seemed also to be a tendency to repeat earlier situations, even painful ones. This tendency to repeat, he believed, acts like a compulsion (i.e., it is an automatic repetitiveness without regard for the reality requirements of the situation). From his observations, it seemed that the tendency to repeat is an attempt either to undo the trauma —by getting back to the time before it happened—or to master it by repeating it. He gave as an example of the attempt at mastery an observation he had made of a child. When the mother went away, the child began a game of hiding a toy and finding it again. Freud concluded that by doing this he denied his helplessness about his mother's going away. In rediscovering his toy, he assured himself that he had control of the situation.[1] A similar attempt at mastery, he thought, may explain the dreams of soldiers. By dreaming of the traumatic situation over and over again, they are attempting to master the emotions produced by the experience.

Following this observation of traumatic neuroses, Freud sought to make a more general application of his theory to neurotic behavior in general. He concluded that the phenomenon of transference fitted very well into the idea of a compulsion to repeat past situations. This would explain its painful as well as its pleasurable aspects. In the transference, the patient repeats his childhood experiences, both good and bad. It was further observed that not only do people tend to repeat earlier life situations in the transference, but there is a general tendency to repeat earlier life patterns over and over again. Thus, for example, a woman may make several unsuccessful marriages. In each, in spite of apparent differences in the personality of the husband and in the general situation, the marriage seems to come to grief in the same way. There seems to be a general automatic repetitiousness of human behavior, especially of neurotic human behavior. This was a very important observation. In brief, the discovery was that the tendency to repeat an earlier situation may be stronger than the pleasure principle.

Consequently, about 1920 Freud had two new observations to add to his theory of instincts: 1. That aggression is not necessarily a product of the libido and yet it can be repressed and be a problem in neurosis; 2. That a tendency to repeat earlier situations explains much of human behavior. Both of

---

[1] Sigmund Freud, *Beyond the Pleasure Principle*, Boni & Liveright, New York, no date, pp. 12-14.

these were important discoveries and much of later theory has been influenced by them. Freud himself developed a new instinct theory which included these two concepts. Sticking to his biological orientation, he sought an explanation comparable to his earlier libido theory. He postulated another instinct—the death instinct—the tendency of organic life to return to the inorganic state whence it came. Both aggression and the tendency to repeat he found related to the death instinct. This idea was congenial to him because it kept intact his theory that the aim of life is to be relieved of tension. The earlier theory is now seen as too limited. The human seeks more than a relief from sexual tension. Living itself involves a state of tension. There is a drive within us which aims always towards death, which is a release of tension.

The new instinct theory again presented a contrasting pair of drives, Eros or the life instinct and the death instinct. Eros is not new. It includes both the old libido and part of the self-preservation (ego) drive. The idea of the death instinct is new. The energy of this instinct is definitely not libido but destructiveness or aggression directed primarily towards the self. It is the force within us which is working towards death. This death instinct Freud now conceived as playing fully as important a part in human life as the libido. The repetition compulsion theoretically is related to the death instinct. It is an expression of the tendency of life to return to earlier states. In the last analysis, this is the tendency of organic life to return to the inorganic.

Sadism must be fitted into this picture. Sadism is produced by combining some of the forces of the death instinct with the libido. This Freud saw as an attempt at self-preservation.

By erotizing some of the destructive forces they become less dangerous to life. The life force tends to neutralize some of their power.

In order to be consistent with the theory of a death instinct, it was necessary to assume that the destructive drive was directed primarily against oneself and was only secondarily turned outwards in aggression towards others. This meant revising his earlier conception of sadism and masochism. He now thought of masochism as the most direct type of union between libido and destructiveness, and sadism as a secondary development, whereas his early idea had been that sadism was primary and masochism was the result of turning sadism against the self.

The problem of life as he now saw it was to keep the self-destructive drive within bounds. This was done either by erotizing it (combining it with libido to form masochism or sadism) or by turning it outwards towards others in aggression. This death instinct turned outwards supplied the drive producing wars. A nation which does not fight, he thought, must destroy itself. Therefore, a war is a nation's attempt at self-preservation. Suicide is seen as evidence of failure to turn the death instinct outward. So are expressions of masochism.

According to the new theory, there are two reasons why we manage to live for many years in spite of our death instinct. One is our ability to turn the energy outward and attack others, and our second protection is the tendency of the life instinct to combine with the death instinct to form masochism. It was assumed that in the combination the two forces tend to neutralize each other, and the destructive drive, for a time at least, becomes less harmful. But it eventually succeeds in "doing" the individual to death.[1]

This is the new instinct theory created by Freud in an attempt to explain clinical observations.

The idea of a death instinct was not accepted with enthusiasm by many of Freud's pupils, although the repetition compulsion and the hypothesis that repressed aggression played an important role in neurosis were readily accepted and applied in therapy.

The concept of a death instinct has certain plausible aspects. It is a fact that complex living organisms tend to die, that in addition to illness and accident, each kind of organism has a fairly definite life cycle. It is at least within the realm of possibility that this life cycle is determined by a drive within the organism. But it has not been proven. This is the basis of Freud's theory; however, it is not what he deals with in applying his theory to patients clinically. There he talks about destructiveness and violence. He assumes that suicide and destructiveness towards others are products of the death instinct. More recent observation by others suggests, however, that they have much more to do with the feeling of being thwarted in living. It is apparent from clinical data that suicide is usually stimulated by motives other than self-destruction. Spite and punishing the "loved" one are almost invariably factors, and it can usually be shown that such drives develop out of interpersonal difficulties.

We have seen before that Freud did not give sufficient weight to the significance of the interplay of the personalities

---

[1] Sigmund Freud, *An Outline of Psychoanalysis*, W. W. Norton & Co., Inc., New York, 1949, p. 23.

of parents and children. Therefore, he attributed the frequent evidence of destructiveness in children to an inherent drive which began to assert itself at the anal stage.

He failed also to note another aspect of the so-called destructiveness of the child: that it is often destructiveness only in terms of adult values. The child breaks things in an inadequate attempt to understand them, or he may break them because he likes the noise. In short, in the pursuit of satisfaction and curiosity he happens to destroy, but destruction is not his goal.

The question must be raised whether this is also true of what looks like deliberate cruelty in children as seen in their torturing of animals and of each other. Certainly some of this cruelty is due to ignorance of the pain induced. If we had adequate statistics, we would probably find that the children who inflict pain with the intention of hurting are children who have been treated cruelly or over-sternly. They are doing, possibly in a more primitive way, what their parents did to them. This, then, would not be the result of a fixed instinct but the result of life experience as it has moulded the raw material of human nature. In short, aggression normally appears in response to frustration. It represents a distortion of the attempt to master life, but cruelty for its own sake probably only occurs as a result of having experienced it from others.

In spite of the complexities of Freud's new instinct theory, it included an important new observation, namely, that when a person's security is threatened, he tends to fight. If he cannot fight because the odds are against him, he tends to become masochistic. That is, in a sense, he rises above the situation by getting a kind of pleasure out of it. These are the clinical observations on which the theory rests. This at last opened new possible sources for understanding the development of hostility and aggression. According to the old theory, hostility and aggression were thought to stem either from the aggressive component of the anal libido or from the feelings of rivalry in the Oedipus situation. There was some general formulation that hate also was an expression of libido. Without repudiating these earlier ideas, the new concept was added.

The questionable point about Freud's theory is the idea that the threat to life and security comes from an innate force within us—destructiveness or the death instinct. If this theory is true, then a child in a perfectly benign environment would nevertheless have a seriously destructive force within himself as a constant menace in need of control. This does not seem to be the case. Serious destructiveness seems to be developed by malevolent environments.

I do not, of course, deny the existence of basic biological drives. My question is rather whether they constitute problems by the very intensity of their energy. The tendency to grow, develop and reproduce seems to be a part of the human organism. When these drives are obstructed by neurotic parents or as a result of a destructive cultural pattern, then the individual develops resentment and hostility either consciously or unconsciously or both. In short, far from being a product of the death instinct, it is an expression of the organism's attempt to live.

Freud's theory of a life and death instinct offered a more comprehensive basis for understanding human behavior than his earlier theory did, but it still sees man as predominantly an instinct-ridden animal and does not give adequate weight to the overwhelming importance of social forces in moulding as well as distorting man's potentialities.

So it can be said that living matter tends to die—there may even be an inherent rhythm about it—but it remains to be proved that there is a connection between this and man's tendency to destructiveness and violence. If these are to be understood, they must rather be dealt with as reactions to being obstructed in living.

Similarly, we may question the validity of Freud's connecting another clinical observation with the death instinct, namely, the repetition compulsion.

Clinically, the discovery of the phenomena to which Freud gave the name repetition compulsion ranks in importance with his earlier discoveries of transference, repression, resistance and unconscious processes. According to the new observation, human behavior is dominated even more powerfully by the tendency to repeat former patterns of life than by the pleasure principle. There seems to be a rigid repetitiveness to life patterns both pleasant and unpleasant. Thus, as illustrated, a girl with a harsh father whom she feared may tend to get herself involved over and over with men of the same type with the same disastrous effect. It is something about which she is apparently powerless. So Freud erroneously concluded it to be a rigid compulsion, and he incorporated it in his instinct theory as a part of the pattern of the death instinct. He believed it to be similar to the tendency of organic matter to return to earlier patterns of inorganic life.

Again, the tendency to connect the "repetition compulsion"

with a biological drive seems to have closed Freud's mind to further observing the actual dynamics of the situation. To him it was a rigid reliving of an earlier situation acting automatically. In transference, for example, the father pattern or mother pattern of early life is superimposed on the analyst, who theoretically does nothing either to merit it or prevent it. It has been found that the phenomena described under the term are more complicated and less rigidly determined than Freud pictured them. He assumed the pattern was fixed by the age of six. No new changes and no new repressions could occur after that. When a new repression seemed to occur in later life, Freud believed it could always be found to be a repetition of an earlier one. If Freud's theory were true, then successful psychoanalytic therapy would be practically impossible.[1]

We agree with Freud that early patterns of behavior, developed in reaction to the personalities of the significant people of our early childhood, are very strong and very important, but some modification of these patterns goes on constantly as the result of experiences with other people throughout childhood and even in adult life.

To take a schematic example—suppose a child developed a submissive attitude in response to a dominating mother. This tendency to be submissive would be used towards all people in authority, but if a teacher, a Boy Scout leader or some other hero of childhood presents a consistently different attitude encouraging the child to assert himself, the original pattern can be considerably altered. If, in addition,

---

[1] In his paper, "Analysis Terminable and Interminable," Freud came substantially to this conclusion.

circumstances offer this child a position of leadership among his contemporaries, he may develop considerable self-assurance and assertiveness. In other words, his original pattern will be definitely changed.

If, on the other hand, the dominating mother is followed by a dominating teacher and the child is so cowed that he shrinks from any leadership and becomes further intimidated by his contemporaries, the personality picture will look like a rigid repetition pattern. The fact is that later life experiences have reinforced the original pattern.

It is easy to see why Freud thought he was dealing with a rigid automatic compulsion. A child finds a way of dealing with the significant adult, his mother. At first she is his total interpersonal experience and he can but assume that this is the way you deal with people and are dealt with, unless a sufficiently different interpersonal experience teaches him otherwise. This is one side of the formation of his pattern. The other aspect is that his attitude stimulates appropriate responses from others. The submissive child, for example, invites domination. That is, by his behavior he invites new people in his environment to treat him as his mother did. He is attractive to and attracted by aggressive people. Thus, the old way of reacting seems to be automatically repeated, but any variation of personality introduced into this picture by some fortunate experience changes the pattern. So the original patterns are the core of subsequent behavior, but this core can be altered constructively or destructively by subsequent life experience. This would mean that the tendency to repeat fairly rigid configurations of behavior is not an innate drive but the product of interpersonal forces. Supposing, for example, a part of a person's emotional attitude is resentment at being "pushed around." The reasonable thing for him to do would be to become self-sufficient so that no one is tempted to push him around. This seldom happens. The most usual experience is that he becomes involved with people who like to dominate, towards whom he reacts with an attitude of helplessness. This is a signal to them to go into action. He then often resentfully thinks this is his fate without being aware of his own contribution to it.

Freud saw this as a pattern acting like a compulsion related to the death instinct. Sullivan and Horney have described it as an evolving process, the result of the interaction of personalities, and in this interaction changes are always being brought about.

Freud's last theory of instincts was definitely an improvement on earlier theories in that it suggested other possible sources of neurosis than the sexual. However, it has the same limitation in perspective as the earlier ones in that it still assumes that man's problem is primarily his struggle with his instincts. By postulating a death instinct, Freud gives self-destructiveness a central place in human life. In so doing, he does not sufficiently distinguish between self-assertion in the interest of growth and self-preservation, and aggression which is not in the interest of anything constructive.

chapter three

THE EGO AND CHARACTER STRUCTURE

WITH THE DISCOVERY OF THE ROLE OF AGGRES sion and the study of repetitive patterns of behavior, the function of the ego eventually became the topic of study. In 1910 Adler made the first move in the direction of stressing the importance of the ego and its functions. Freud, as we have seen, had earlier assumed that ego drives were not subject to repression and therefore played no part in neurosis. He repudiated Adler's work on the basis that in stressing ego traits he was denying the importance of the unconscious and was, therefore, no longer dealing with the material of psychoanalysis.[1] Freud at the time certainly failed to see a fact which became clear to him in the 1920's, that ego drives might also be unconscious. So Adler's discovery made no impression on the main stream of psychoanalysis.

However, soon after 1910, Freud began to give some consideration to the ego. In 1911 he wrote a very important paper on "Two Principles of Mental Functioning" in which,

---

[1] For Freud at this time unconscious material was always related to libid inal drives.

while stressing again his already well established theory that the libido functioned according to the pleasure principle, he pointed out that ego drives seemed more under the influence of the reality principle. Out of the necessity of comprehending reality developed man's ability to observe, remember and think. In short, out of the need to cope with reality grew the ego as we know it. Ferenczi,[1] in 1913, elaborated the theme in his paper, "Stages in the Development of the Sense of Reality." He showed that in the process of growth, not only the libido went through stages; the ego also came only gradually to full comprehension of its function of reality testing.

He suggested that the ego emerges gradually, going through four preliminary stages before clearly becoming differentiated as an entity. The first stage is the period of "unconditional omnipotence." This is the situation of the child before birth when all wishes are gratified. Immediately after birth is the period of "magic hallucinatory omnipotence." At this time, he thought, the infant must feel that he only needs to wish something and it is there. As his needs become more complex, there are times of disappointment, but then he discovers that by cries and gestures he can produce results. This is the period of "omnipotence by magic gestures." And finally comes the stage of power through "magic thoughts and words." Gradually the feeling of omnipotence fades, although Ferenczi suggested that some people never give up the idea of magic and keep the illusion of power in the idea of free will.

At any rate, the ego and its function were beginning to be

[1] Sandor Ferenczi, *Sex in Psychoanalysis*, Ch. VIII.

noted. As has already been mentioned, the discovery of the importance of repressed aggression further focused attention on the ego. In the early 1920's Freud finally formulated a theory of the total personality, and the ego with its function of reality testing became the Ego of the Ego, Superego and Id.

Freud saw the newborn infant as chiefly Id, that is, masses of impulses without an organizing or directing consciousness. Contact with the world gradually modifies a portion of this Id and a small area of consciousness, the Ego, slowly emerges from it. It is developed out of the necessity for reality testing. However, the Ego is not synonymous with consciousness. Only a small part even of the Ego is conscious at any one time. A great part of the Ego as now defined exists outside of awareness but can readily be called into awareness when needed. This part was called the preconscious. Still another part of the Ego is unconscious and cannot readily be made conscious. This consists of the experiences and feelings which have been repressed. These experiences, by the fact of their repression, are somehow brought into more intimate contact with the forces of the Id.

The Id is a mass of seething excitement which cannot become conscious directly. Many of its forces never reach awareness, but from time to time portions of its energy can find some expression in the Ego by becoming connected with the memory-traces of repressed experience and thus participating in the formation of symptoms; becoming distorted as in dream symbols; or by undergoing modification chiefly as a result of the influence of the Superego as in sublimation. The Id Freud conceived of as of tremendous size in comparison with the Ego. He thought of it as the generator of energy,

the dynamo of the personality. It is somehow closely associated with the organic processes of the body.

In the course of time, the Ego takes over certain standards
from the culture, chiefly through the influence of training by
parents in early childhood. These standards become incorporated as parent images within the Ego as a part of itself
and this part is called the Superego. It exercises a criticizing
and censoring power. The functions of dream censor and resistance described in Freud's earlier writings are now seen as
part of the Superego. The Superego, in brief, represents the
incorporated standards of society. It includes the parental attitudes, especially as these attitudes were understood and
interpreted by the child in his early years. It includes also
the person's own ideals for himself, and Freud even indicates
that certain phylogenetic experiences such as those described
by Jung under the concept of the collective unconscious may
also be part of the Superego. Much of the Superego is unconscious because it was incorporated by the child very early
and without his awareness. This means that like all unconscious material this portion is not available for reality testing. This partially accounts for the irrational harshness of
some of the attitudes of a man's conscience towards his behavior. For example, it may make him feel guilty about an
act for which he consciously has no feelings of regret. Freud
further attributes some of the harshness of the Superego to a
theoretical relation to the death instinct. This is too complicated to be discussed here.[1] The Superego is an important
construction. It is, in effect, Freud's way of talking about in-

---

[1] Sigmund Freud, *Civilization and Its Discontents*, Jonathan Cape & Harrison Smith, New York, 1930, Ch. 7.

terpersonal relations, and the influence of the culture on man's behavior.

The Ego, as Freud saw it, holds an executive position. Its function is to reconcile the Id, the Superego and the outside world. It must permit the Id to let off enough steam so that its forces are not a dangerous threat and yet not offend the Superego or run afoul of the outside world. It is, so to speak, the master of compromise. With the aid of the Superego, it makes the forces of the Id harmless by forming sublimations or reaction formations from them.

Character structure, as Freud saw it, is the result of subli- mation or reaction formation. That is, it is formed uncon- sciously through the efforts of the Superego to bind the forces of the Id in such a way that the Ego accepts them, and its relation to the outside world is not jeopardized. It is, in effect, a defensive mechanism. Although the result, sublima- tion, seems to be a positive attitude of the Ego, it is formed primarily as a defense against instincts. Freud's philosophy of character makes it the result of the transformation of in- stinctual drives.

The concept of the individual described in *The Ego and the Id* is, as Freud himself says, merely a theoretical construc- tion which may or may not have validity, but it had a far reaching practical result. In this work (*The Ego and the Id*) Freud for the first time shifted his interest from the libido to the activities of the Ego. This shift influenced the technique of therapy. Within a few years, analysts were to become less concerned with what happens to the libido and very much concerned with the ways in which the Ego defends itself. The analysis of character structure was a direct outcome of the new interest. In the late 1920's Wilhelm Reich was already teaching new methods for dealing with the complicated defenses of the Ego, and most of the discoveries of recent years relate to the unconscious processes of the Ego.

Ideas about the nature of character began to be formulated in 1908. True to the particular bent of psychoanalysis, Freud saw character in terms of libido. *Character,* as used in psychoanalysis, is a term applied to a relatively permanent constellation of characteristics or habitual attitudes. It should not be confused here with its meaning in popular language. In recent years, Fromm has made a further distinction between temperament and character. Temperament is defined as something constitutional. For example, some people are more placid than others, some more vigorous, some more high-strung. These may be innate differences recognizable from the time of birth. The term character, in psychoanalysis, is used only for habitual attitudes developed as reactions to life situations. Possibly temperament has something to do with determining the character direction chosen by a given person, but the character is something in addition to temperament. For example, a phlegmatic person may in addition develop a passive character pattern and a vigorous, energetic type may become domineering.

All people, of course, have some form of character structure. These are their habitual ways of reacting to the world; possibly there are somewhat different ways of reacting to superiors, to inferiors, to friends and enemies, but underlying all the variations each person has a characteristic way, in general, of meeting life. Symptoms might be considered special aspects of character trends in that symptoms are consistent with the character. Thus, one seldom finds a washing compulsion in a happy-go-lucky, generous person. A washing compulsion seems more frequently to be related to a suspicious, withdrawn, pessimistic way of looking at life.

Freud in 1908 first presented a theory of character structure. It was not until nearly twenty years later that a successful therapeutic approach to the problem was worked out by others.

Freud's first paper on the subject was entitled "Character and Anal Eroticism." The theory here presented, that a character has its origin in the libido, is still today the theory accepted in classical analysis. Fromm, Sullivan and Horney have formulated other methods of character formation, which will be discussed presently.

According to Freud, in the formation of character one of three things may happen to the libido. A part of the libido of any pregenital stage of development may continue unchanged into adult life. The result of such a course was termed a perversion and was thought to be not a true character development. The two other possibilities were the development of reaction formations against the instinct and sublimations of the instinct. These last two methods accounted for character, and it was believed that these were the ways in which human beings matured. Since man was thought of as essentially a creature of his libido, he became a social being by the process of reaction formation and sublimation. What was meant by this was first described in the 1908 paper in connection with anal libido.

Those who without sublimation keep their anal interests through life continue to show a childish pleasure in feces and

anal sensations. This, Freud stated, was especially characteristic of passive homosexuals and is not a true character
formation.

Another group with a strong fixation on anal interests
shows a tendency to develop reaction formations against the
instincts. This usually appears as great orderliness and neatness. It pertains not only to bodily cleanliness but to reliabil-
ity and conscientiousness, especially about petty duties.

The solution by sublimation is seen best exemplified in the
attitude towards money. Pleasure in the feces becomes sublimated in pleasure in money. The child's feeling of power
in controlling his feces becomes the feeling of power in the
manipulation of money. The extreme character development
here would be the miser. Parsimonious and stingy people
also have anal characters, and even the sharp businessman
has "anal" traits.

Another type of sublimation of anal libido has to do with
pleasure in handling feces. This, according to Freud, accounts for the sculptor and painter, who manipulate objects
and materials. Less directly it might relate to pleasure in
most manual crafts.

As a matter of practical experience, the distinction between sublimation and reaction formation is not always completely clear. Theoretically, in reaction formation the denial
of the instinctual pleasure dominates the picture, while in
sublimation the instinctual gratification supposedly finds some
expression. Thus, the antivivisectionist is denying his sadism,
and the surgeon is supposedly enjoying his sadism in a socially useful way.

According to Freud's theory, in the formation of character the actual libidinal energy becomes bound and utilized in the character trait.

His first paper on character, although very short, presented all the essential points for a complete theory of the way character is formed. Later writers, especially Jones and Abraham, elaborated the anal character further, but there was no disagreement with Freud. There is no doubt that the personality pattern described exists, although not always in the pure state. The questioning of recent writers is as to whether it is the product of anal libido.

Freud described the anal character as showing orderliness, parsimony and obstinacy. In the history of these cases, he said, there is always found difficulty in learning to control the bowels. There is a tendency to hold back and resist becoming regular in bowel movements. When this problem is finally overcome, the character traits appear. Therefore, he concluded, toilet difficulties have been replaced by character traits. Apparently the fact that the character traits seemed to appear at the point of mastering toilet difficulties was considered sufficient proof that the one was transformed into the other. No further proof was presented.

Jones and Abraham wrote more at length of the anal character, accepting Freud's hypothesis without question. Abraham described the anal character as a type of personality inaccessible, withdrawn, stubborn, generally hostile and methodical in an obsessional way. It is a thorough, meticulous but unproductive character. The tendency to save everything is marked. People with an anal character are not only misers with money, but they fear wasting time and cannot throw anything away. This kind of character is the most thoroughly studied of the Freudian types.

Five other types of character based on fixation at various stages of libido development have been described by classical Freudians, Abraham [1] making the chief contribution. In each the characteristic attitudes are assumed to be reaction formations or sublimations of the libido of the stage under discussion. The oral receptive is considered a sublimation of the earliest sucking stage of life. When it is a positive sublimation, these people are characterized by friendliness, optimism and generosity. They always expect things to turn out right but make very little effort to bring it about. They expect the whole world to mother them. The generosity is due to wanting to give others also the feeling that everything will turn out well, and they will be cared for. They are not hostile and their attitude towards others is friendly and positive in contrast to the anal character, who is suspicious and withdrawn.

When persons with an oral character are frustrated, they are pessimists who act as if the bottom had fallen out of the world. The oral character must always be surrounded by people. He cannot endure solitude.

The second oral stage, as described by Abraham, is believed to be a sublimation of the biting stage, which develops as the result of the appearance of teeth. These are people who are aggressive and exploit others. They, so to speak, rend and tear off what they want from life. Envy and ambition are important in their make-up.

[1] Karl Abraham, *Selected Papers on Psychoanalysis*, The Hogarth Press, Ltd., London, 1927, Chapters 12, 23, 24, 25.

A phallic character [1] comes from sublimation of the phallic stage. Such a person is, among other things, insolent, domineering, and aggressive.

A urethral character has also been mentioned by Freud and Ferenczi very briefly. Burning ambition and a need to boast of achievement are outstanding traits in this type. They are impatient people and there is usually a history of bedwetting beyond the usual age.

A mature or genital type of character is described by Abraham. It supposedly is developed in the same way as the others by sublimation of or reaction formation against sexual drives not permitted direct gratification. Since Freud believed that civilization was developed at the expense of the sexual drive, one should assume that the most mature people are those who have renounced the most. Abraham sees genital characters as people no longer dominated by the pleasure principle. While people in all other stages are narcissistic, these are not. They are friendly, loving and demonstrate elements of the preceding stages in proportions conducive to the most effectiveness. That is, they are receptive, sufficiently self-assertive to make a place for themselves and show an adequate degree of caution and foresight. Fromm notes that the mature character also has a new trait—the capacity to give and to care for the welfare of another. It should be noted that Fromm, in discussing these types, does not subscribe to their libido origin. He points out that Freud's character types each represent an important attitude towards assimilation. By assimilation Fromm means the process of coping with the

[1] Wilhelm Reich, *Character Analysis*, Orgone Institute Press, New York, 1945, Ch. 10, Section 3.

particular life situation, including the acquiring of knowledge and skills and making them a part of oneself. Freud, especially as interpreted by Abraham, explains them in terms of libido. Abraham's assumption is that the oral receptive character met with significant experiences at the oral stage or possibly had a constitutional predisposition to oral interests. The anal character had similar experiences at the anal stage, etc.

These basic character types of classical analysis do not exhaust the descriptive possibilities. One hears of obsessional characters, narcissistic characters, hysterical characters, etc. These are names from other frames of reference and stress specific aspects of the basic types. The obsessional character is a form of anal character where the obsessional quality is predominant. The narcissistic character includes all types except the mature genital character. The hysterical character seems to be a combination of the oral aggressive and phallic.

In summary, classical analysis has two general types of character classification. One stresses the libido origin. These are oral, anal, phallic, urethral, and genital. The other type of classification is in terms of the clinical picture and includes the narcissistic, hysterical and obsessional or compulsive.

From the description, it is apparent that Freud and his immediate followers hoped to solve the problem of character along the same lines as that of neurosis and symptoms. That is, it was a question of understanding the distribution of libido. There is no doubt that as clinical descriptions of people and their ways of mastering life they are important, but we should look carefully at the theory of their origin. We must question whether it is a fact that the very orderly person is one who had difficulty in becoming anally clean and possibly had more pleasure than the average in soiling himself, that the oral receptive type had significant experience in sucking and the oral aggressive had especially important biting experiences. The postulating of a libido origin for character is misleading. To a large extent it leaves out of consideration the overwhelming influence of the parents in moulding the child's personality. Reich, Anna Freud and Alexander, like Freud and Abraham, nevertheless saw character in terms of libido.

A theory of character in non-libidinal terms was first presented by Jung in his Psychological Types. He made two major divisions of people—the introvert and the extravert. The introvert turns in upon himself, is absorbed in his inner world, while the extravert turns outward to the world, and is much more concerned with what goes on there than with his own private experiences. Both of these types he subdivides into thinking, feeling, intuition and sensation types. That is, there may be a thinking introvert, a thinking extravert, a feeling introvert or extravert and so on. The ways in which these characters are developed requires a more thorough exposition of Jung's system than is the function of this chapter.

The next person to present a classification of character types was Rank. Oriented around his concept of the role of will, he divided people into the normal (adjusted), the neurotic and the creative artist. The normal person is the one who has surrendered his will and accepted the will of the group. The neurotic is the person who cannot conform to the will of the group and yet is not free to assert his own will and be a creative artist. His neurosis is his work of art. The creative artist is the one who affirms his own will. Neither Jung's nor Rank's frame of reference readily lend themselves to comparison of their character types with the Freudian classification. There is, however, some similarity between Rank's types and Fromm's later formulations. The normal or adjusted person corresponds roughly with the marketing personality of Fromm (to be discussed later) in that in the description of both, conformity to the will and goals of the group is the basic premise. One should note here that "adjustment" is not necessarily mental health. One may conform out of fear of disapproval or for other reasons; in some cultures conformity may be against one's own best interests. The creative artist of Rank has some points in common with Fromm's productive character, but certain ways in which it is described make its maturity somewhat open to question. For example, as will be shown when Rank is considered in more detail, he thought of the creative artist as making his own "truth." This could mean that he is mature enough no longer to need to lean on the authority of others to confirm the rightness of his actions, but it could also mean that he is a law unto himself and that a thing is good because he wills it to be to the exclusion of the rights of others. The latter would certainly be far from a mature person.

Of the so-called cultural school of analysts, Fromm has written more specifically of character structure than either Horney or Sullivan. In his character types—receptive, exploitative and hoarding—there is a new presentation of the character patterns described by Abraham as oral receptive, oral aggressive and anal. Fromm, however, has a new conception of their origins. Instead of seeing them as the result of libido sublimation, he sees them as basic attitudes in the process of assimilation and socialization. In his opinion, character types are the product of the interaction of child and parent. In one type of home, a child develops the attitude of expecting to receive because the situation under the circumstances is best manipulated by being receptive, friendly and pleasing. In a more frustrating atmosphere, the child may feel he can have only what he takes, that the only source of security is in exploiting others. If the home atmosphere is ungiving, anxious and suspicious, the child will be impressed with a "feeling of scarcity" and may well develop the "anal" characteristic of hanging on to what he has because there may not be any more. The parental influences are effective from the first moment of life and the child's character begins to be formed at that point.

In connection with his thesis, Fromm asks the question: if the so-called anal character has nothing to do with anal libido, why are such people usually constipated? Why are oral characters fond of eating and drinking? He concludes that constipation and love of eating are not causes of character formation but expressions of it. The stingy person hangs on to everything, including his feces. He is not stingy because he hangs on to feces, and he may or may not have had difficulty in childhood with constipation. In general, the type of parent who withholds tends to have a meticulous attitude towards toilet training. Such a mother is not capable of being indulgent of a child's toilet whims any more than she can be indulgent about anything else. Already in nursing rules, the same ungiving attitude will be present. More "permissive" parents, on the other hand, enjoy seeing their children eat. So, to a child in such a home, receiving food may well be a symbol of receiving from a friendly world.

Fromm also adds a fourth type of character under his non-productive orientations. This he calls the marketing personality, which he considers especially characteristic of this culture. Briefly, it is a type of character oriented to market value. "I am as you desire me" is the dominating attitude. In short, the person is opportunistically oriented.

A fifth type is the productive character. Here the outstanding characteristic is the capacity for love and creative work. This type differs from the others in having predominantly positive attributes. Fromm's productive character, like Abraham's genital character, may contain qualities remaining from the earlier stages, but they would be under the dominance of the productive orientation; in no case would he have the undesirable traits. Thus receptiveness would be expressed here as adaptability, exploitativeness becomes ability to take initiative, etc.

Fromm states that "the process of living implies two kinds of relatedness to the outside world, that of assimilation and that of socialization." [1] The types already described are related to assimilation. In the process of socialization, he describes more specifically the characteristic ways of interacting with people. These are by symbiotic relatedness, withdrawal, destructiveness and love. In symbiotic relatedness, dependency on another person is outstanding. One may either "swallow" the other person or be "swallowed." Often the dependency is benevolent but it can be cruel.

Withdrawal or destructiveness are traits of those who seek

[1] *Man for Himself*, p. 107.

their security by isolation. The withdrawal may be conscious or unconscious. In the latter case, the indifference may be concealed under a superficial affability. Destructiveness is a more active trait. The other person is seen as so dangerous that he must be destroyed.

Love is defined by Fromm as the productive form of relatedness. It does not manipulate the other person but shows respect and responsibility for him and the desire to see him grow and develop.

Horney does not specifically speak of character types but her descriptions of neurotic trends, as methods of avoiding anxiety, actually amount to character syndromes. Horney describes three general ways of reacting—moving towards people, moving against and moving away. These would correspond, in general, with Fromm's symbiotic relatedness (moving towards), destructiveness (moving against) and withdrawal (moving away).

Sullivan's description of personality types cannot readily be compared with the concept of character developed by the Freudian school. His theory of the self-system, however, includes an explanation of the development of habitual attitudes, and thus definitely concerns itself with the same aspects of a person descriptively speaking. The dynamics are, however, quite different. It is difficult to make an adequate comparison at this time without discussing Sullivan's theories at length (see Chapter 10).

Briefly, the self-system consists of a configuration of traits which have mainly met with the approval of significant people, especially in childhood.[1] Generally, attributes which

[1] The exceptions will be discussed in Chapter 10.

meet with disapproval tend to be blocked out of awareness and are not a part of the self-system except as they sometimes gain access to it in disguised form through sublimation. Here Sullivan uses the word sublimation without subscribing to Freud's definition of it as the transformation of libido.

The self-system of Sullivan has this in common with Freud's concept of character: it is formed as a result of the influence of the parents on the developing personality of the child. Freud presents this idea more mechanistically when he says character is the result of the sublimation of instincts under the influence of the Superego, the Superego being mainly the incorporated attitudes of the parents and society. The self-system is different from the concept of character in that it includes more than sublimation, whereas Freud seems to conceive of character as nothing but sublimation. No true comparison of the two can be made because the frames of reference are entirely different. Freud's system emphasizes what happens to instincts. Sullivan's system stresses what goes on between people. For Sullivan personality does not develop mechanically. Always the emphasis is on a dynamic interaction between people. Freud's orientation is mechanistic-biological; Sullivan's dynamic-cultural (interpersonal).

As has already been pointed out, it took many years from the inception of interest in character to a practical application of the findings to therapy. In many ways the theories are chiefly of academic interest. In psychology in general there seems to be a temptation to put people in classes, and these analytically oriented attempts are not the only examples to be found.

However, understanding of character as described in psychoanalysis eventually has proved of value in therapy. The defenses which an individual develops against gaining insight into his difficulties are always consistent with his character structure. He acts as if he had a stake in maintaining this structure unaltered. The cause of the rigidity about this is well described by Sullivan (see Chapter 10). The way it works in therapy is as follows. The receptive type of person, for instance, when confronted with danger, by his friendliness disarms his adversary. The hoarding type withdraws and refuses "to give out." The exploiting type tries to manipulate the situation by flattery, aggression or other means. As long as the characteristic ways of coping with people are able to function in dealing with the analyst, the patient experiences no anxiety and also gains no insight. This constitutes the type of obstacle presented by the character and Reich was the first person to see it clearly. This will be presented in more detail in discussing transference.

It is obvious that the study of character structure as it relates to therapy is a relatively recent development in psychoanalysis. Certainly there is still much more to learn about it. Whatever theory in the long run proves to be most adequate, one thing has been accomplished to date. By establishing the idea that the habitual attitudes provide the resistance to cure, a new era in treatment has begun. No longer is the drive to unearth the past paramount in therapy. The way the person defends himself in his daily relations with people has become the main object of study, although his past history is also examined in order to provide insight as to how he got to be the sort of person he is.

chapter four

UNCONSCIOUS PROCESSES AND REPRESSION

THE LIBIDO THEORY AND THE INSTINCT THEORIES developed on the basis of the libido concept have so permeated the thinking of psychoanalysis that one is in danger of assuming that all of Freud's discoveries are related to and dependent upon them.

The fact is that Freud's earliest discoveries were made before he elaborated a sexual theory of neurosis, and the importance and validity of these earliest observations far outweighs any later theorizing. His bringing to light the fact that a part of a person's life goes on outside awareness, that this unconscious part influences experience and behavior, and his study of the way things become unconscious and are kept so are among his greatest contributions. Also the discovery of that phenomenon in the doctor-patient relationship to which he gave the name transference was the beginning of the understanding of another very important aspect of human behavior.

Although there are evidences of some awareness of unconscious processes before the time of Breuer and Freud—and this vague knowledge was utilized in hypnosis—there was no systematic investigation of them and no attempt to work out their relation to mental disorder, or human experience and behavior in general. The studies of Breuer and Freud were the beginning of research out of which was to grow the whole system of theory and therapy of psychoanalysis.

That a part of a person's life experience might become unconscious was the first discovery noted and elaborated. In 1880 Breuer was treating a patient, Anna O., by hypnosis. She was suffering from multiple hysterical manifestations and, as was the fashion of the day, Breuer was attempting to remove the symptoms by suggestion under hypnosis. In this case something unusual happened. Under light hypnosis the patient began to talk of events of her past life about which she apparently had no memory in her "waking" state. Moreover, it soon became apparent that these memories had some sort of relation to her symptoms because after talking of the memories the symptoms disappeared. One example will illustrate. The patient had a hysterical paralysis of one arm. It was revealed in the hypnoid state that this related to a specific memory. The girl had been caring for her father who was fatally ill. One night while she was sitting by his bedside waiting for the arrival of a specialist from a distant city, she apparently dozed with her arm over the back of the chair. In her half waking state she had a dream or hallucination of a snake coming out of the wall towards her father. She tried to reach the snake and then it seemed that her arm was the snake. When she fully roused herself she found her arm was asleep. Breuer concluded that this was the memory which seemed to have later found expression in the paralyzed arm, for after she had recalled it the paralysis vanished. He, at the time, thought of this experience only as a painful memory in the conventional sense. He stressed the girl's concern over her father's welfare as the important factor. However, with our more extensive knowledge today, it is apparent that the situation was quite complicated, that not only was there concern for the father, but there were also negative aspects to her feeling about him.

Still even with the rudimentary understanding of the 1880's, Breuer from many similar observations came to the conclusion that in hysteria symptoms were produced by the shutting off from consciousness of painful memories. These, he saw, were not forgotten in the sense that they no longer existed, but they seemed to continue to exert an influence and finally found expression in symptoms. He concluded that the memory must continue to exist in a dissociated state and that the fact that it was not conscious in some way gave it its pathological power.

Freud, during the 1880's, became a pupil of Breuer and together they made further observations. At first it was thought that the phenomenon later called repression was only found in cases of hysteria, but a few years later Freud demonstrated that the same dissociation could explain dreams and slips of speech and that something similar occurred in obsessional neurosis and phobias. So he postulated that in everybody it is possible for thoughts and life experiences to exist outside conscious awareness. It has been noted that the fact that the first discoveries were made through the study of hysterical symptoms to some extent may account for Freud's conclusion that sex was the most important etiological factor in neurosis. In addition the pattern of hysteria may also have left another mark on the direction of theoretical speculation. Since its symptoms appear as somatic manifestations, this placed emphasis on the idea that somatic processes, specifically sexual energy processes, seemed to be the material involved.

At any rate, in the early 1890's Breuer and Freud came to the following three conclusions about hysteria. A hysterical symptom represents a forgotten memory or condensation of several. Secondly the forgotten memory is in some way expressed by the symptom. It may be expressed symbolically as, for example, nausea may express moral disgust, or a part of the forgotten event may become the symbol of the whole experience as was the case of the paralyzed arm in the example already described. The third conclusion was that no hysterical symptom exists without a forgotten memory.

Breuer and Freud each had a different theory as to what produced the forgetting. Breuer's theory was that certain conditions favored dissociation. States of fatigue, states on the edge of sleep, monotonous employment such as sewing, caring for the sick, were situations creating a kind of twilight state. Monotonous employment was thought to encourage twilight states because it encouraged the development of daydreaming and this made one less aware of what was going on in his immediate environment. Because he was not fully conscious, the person then seemed to be especially vulnerable. Breuer called these states hypnoid states and believed that disturbing experiences happening during them tended to be walled off from consciousness. Freud was not satisfied with this theory. He felt something more than an accidental state of mind was necessary, that a thing must become unconscious for a reason. He believed a thought or memory must be actively put out of the mind because, for some reason, it is unbearable. Thus, he concluded, an act of will is required to make an experience unconscious, and he called the process repression.

Briefly, Breuer's theory was that a thing became unconscious because of the accidental mental state of the patient, while Freud thought there was always a motive for forgetting. Both agreed that the state of being outside awareness accounted for the pathological difficulty. Because of being dissociated, the emotions connected with the event could not be adequately discharged and could not be assimilated by the rest of the personality. Therefore, they concluded that their cures had been due to making the forgotten memory conscious and thus relating it to the rest of the personality so that its energy could be discharged and the experience could be assimilated.

The problem then was to find a way of making unconscious material conscious. In this hypnosis had been effective in the case of Anna O. and others, but some patients could not be hypnotized. It was in the course of an unsuccessful attempt at hypnosis that Freud's patient revealed a method which was to become the basic technique of psychoanalysis. This patient, although she did not go into a hypnotic state and apparently remained fully conscious, acted in the way hypnotized subjects did. She allowed her thoughts to flow freely and reported uncritically everything that went through her mind. In the course of the recital, she reacted with adequate emotion to the thoughts she was expressing. Thus *free association* was discovered, and it was soon apparent that it had an advantage over hypnosis in that the patient remained conscious and did not have to be informed later of what had taken place. This early method of cure was likened to a catharsis. It was believed that simply getting the material out accomplished the cure. The process was called *abreaction*. Thus Freud discovered the existence of repression, the ability to put unbearable memories out of the conscious mind, and he established abreaction through free association as a means of undoing the process of repression.

Freud first used the term repression in the limited sense of an active putting something out of consciousness. It was assumed that the experience had been conscious at least for a brief moment. Later the term was used more generally. As early as 1894 he speaks of a form of dissociation which occurs because the ideas or emotions are not permitted in the social milieu. These dissociated feelings, he thought, had never been conscious, therefore had not been repressed (as he defined the term at that time); yet they seemed able to produce symptoms also. This situation was especially the case with thoughts and feelings which were unacceptable in the social milieu and where the prohibition against them had happened so early in life that probably in most cases they had never verbally been brought to a person's attention. As time went on, this was also called repression and, in fact, all methods of keeping thoughts and feelings unconscious were for many years referred to as repression. In *The Problem of Anxiety* in the 1920's, Freud again reverted to the earlier, more specific definition of repression and listed it as only one of the forms of defense utilized by the Ego. He listed eight others of equal importance—regression, reaction formation, isolation, undoing, projection, introjection, turning against the self, and reversal. Anna Freud in 1936 pointed out that sublimation also was a defense. These later distinctions are of theoretical interest in that they more precisely define the different mechanisms used in bringing about dissociation. But analysts today still generally use repression as a kind of blanket term to include all of the methods of producing dissociation.

The theories about unconscious processes and repression were first worked out in connection with hysteria. Freud soon found that something similar happened in obsessional neurosis and phobias and that probably also psychosis was produced by a comparable method. The first type of repression, that of actively putting out of the mind, seemed to be the usual one with single traumatic episodes, while the second type, where the situation had never been conscious, would occur with more insidiously developing difficulties. The second type of repression would be characteristic of the character defenses which were not understood in the early years. The first type was especially frequent in hysteria.

The purpose of repression as first understood was the avoidance of pain. In the case of Anna O. there is no emphasis on a sexual factor. It was not long before Freud concluded that a sexual factor must always be a part of the painful situation. Probably the general attitude of insincerity about the sexual life characteristic of the Victorian era contributed greatly to drawing Freud's attention to it in that, because it was a forbidden topic, patients were especially prone to repress their thoughts in connection with the subject. Soon frightening sexual experiences were noted as the usual repressed material and eventually there developed the increasing emphasis on sexual drives already discussed. The emphasis on sexual drives in turn had a great influence on Freud's evolving theories of unconscious processes. Unconscious came to be more and more visualized as a place where the instincts or their mental surrogates resided.[1] And so finally appeared the Id, "a chaos, a cauldron of seething excitement . . . there is nothing corresponding to the idea of time . . . the Id knows no values, no good and evil, no morality." [2] In other words, by 1920 "unconscious" had become "the unconscious," a place with definite characteristics. To be sure, Freud stated that this was but a figure of speech and said that he could not allocate any area in the body as the specific province of the Id. Nevertheless, one gets the impression that the idea of *the unconscious* as a place appealed to him and that he thought it possible that some day such an area would be found.

I shall now elaborate in more detail the process of development of the theory. Since the early observations of the working of repression were made in connection with hysteria, the first idea about the condition of an unconscious thought or memory was that it is pretty completely encapsulated, that is, it is almost entirely shut off from any influence on the rest of the personality. It may conceivably remain permanently outside of awareness unless a special kind of subsequent event or life situation succeeds in disturbing it. When that

---

[1] Sigmund Freud, *New Introductory Lectures*, W. W. Norton & Co., Inc., New York, 1933, p. 102. ". . . the word *unconscious* has more and more been made to mean a mental province rather than a quality which mental things have."

[2] *New Introductory Lectures*, pp. 104-105.

occurs, it directly erupts to the surface in the form of a hysterical symptom. According to this theory a person may, for instance, develop hysterical paralysis but otherwise remain "normal." Since we have gained more knowledge of character structure, it has become clear that this is not the case, that probably every repression constantly influences the total personality, and that the formation of a symptom is only one evidence of its effect.

Freud also believed that repression could only occur in early childhood. If a repression seemed to happen later, it was because the situation was directly associated with an early childhood repression which now was re-activated. Here more recent workers would disagree. There is no evidence to prove that there is a specific age beyond which new traumatic experiences cannot be dealt with by repression. A sufficiently traumatic experience in adult life such as war experiences and the torture experiences of concentration camps, for example, conceivably can produce repression without postulating an earlier similar experience. The kernel of truth in Freud's thinking is that a child is more vulnerable than an adult and that unfortunate experiences in childhood produce sufficient personality handicap to make such a person as an adult more vulnerable in the presence of further difficulty or disaster.

Very early in his work with patients, Freud became convinced that every repression would be found to have a sexual core, and he concluded that only the frustration of sexual impulses could produce repression. Later, as we have already seen, he included aggression as another impulse contributing to repression.

The stressing of the sexual (instinct) nature of repressed material had certain unfortunate consequences. It turned attention from the more dynamic situational (interpersonal) aspect of repression and placed the emphasis on the *content* of repression. Interest centered not so much in what life experience produced this, but how an instinct became related to the repression.

Also, the theory that instincts were always involved strengthened the idea of *the* unconscious as a place. Since instincts are a part of the biological endowment, they must reside somewhere. Thus came the idea of the Id, the home of the instincts, and Freud visualized the unconscious as having "topographical" features consisting of three parts, the Id, the repressed part of the Ego, and a part of the repressing agent iself, that is, a part of the Superego.[1] This picture of a place containing all three elements was responsible for the idea that the fact of becoming unconscious somehow throws the content of repression into contact with the instincts, which now, through the repressed memories, can find a means of influencing the Ego. Since both repressed experiences and Id forces are exerting a constant pressure towards outward expression, he thought, they may join forces, that is, the repressed material may borrow some of the energy of the Id to aid it in forcing an outlet. Of course, the highly speculative aspect of this is the idea that the act of repressing brings an experience into contact with the instincts. If we accept it as a hypothesis, it is difficult to see how to start collecting evidence of its validity, since the working of instinct

[1] Of course, the conscious aspects of the personality are also included in this "topographical" scheme.

in the human being is especially difficult to detect. A more fruitful field of research is the study of the relation of the repressed to the repressing force. Here at least we deal with phenomena which can be observed. This, the object of Freud's early interest, was later neglected by him, but several writers of recent years have turned again to a study of the dynamics of repression. This leads away from the concept of *the* unconscious, a place, and stresses once more, as in the earlier thinking, the more fluid interchange between conscious and unconscious processes.

As has been indicated, because of the isolated, somewhat encapsulated nature of repression in hysteria, the impression was first conveyed that when a memory becomes unconscious it has been completely walled off and has no influence on the general personality unless a subsequent event reactivates it. In obsessions the procedure is not so simple, and here Freud recognized that only part of the experience is repressed, that sometimes, for example, the memory of an experience remains in consciousness, but there is no longer any adequate feeling connected with it. When character defenses became the object of study, the relative nature of unconsciousness became more apparent. It was recognized that encapsulated repressions could occur but most of the significant material presented by patients showed widely varying degrees of awareness or unawareness, and these variations were especially apparent in the reactions of a person to different people. This has been especially well demonstrated by Sullivan.[1] A person may reveal certain aspects of himself and his rela-

[1] Harry Stack Sullivan, "Introduction to the Study of Interpersonal Relations," *Psychiatry*, Vol. I, 1938, pp. 121-134.

tionships to one person and quite other aspects to another. In fact there occurs some variation in every interpersonal situation. This applies not only to conscious modifications of behavior to suit the circumstances, but there also occurs unconscious adaptation to the presence of the other person. All sets of reactions to all people are consistent with a general personality pattern, but the total configuration of traits is never called out in any one situation. The part of the personality coming into play with each person is determined by the specific interaction of the two personalities on each other.

An illustration will make this clearer. A patient whose general attitude in analysis was one of docile acceptance, who readily agreed with all interpretations suggested and seemed to have no resentment or doubts, came one day with the following dream.

She had gone to a surgeon about her dizziness. He had undertaken an operation on her brain under local anesthetic. During the operation she realized from his conversation with his assistants that he did not know what he was doing. There was a feeling of horror at his irresponsibility. After the operation the surgeon broke the news to her in a heartless way that she would never walk again.

The patient professed to be greatly amused by the dream, saying jokingly that it looked as if I were right that she did not trust me. When I insisted upon her taking the situation seriously and pointed out that it must mean that she had serious doubts of me, she finally said that she did not like the color of my living room wall. More hesitantly, she admitted she wished I would reduce, but nothing further occurred to her. She talked of other subjects. Suddenly after twenty minutes, she remembered that she had heard a disparaging comment the day before about a paper of mine. This had disturbed her greatly, so much so that she felt she must be sure not to mention it to another patient of mine with whom she was having dinner because it might destroy his confidence in me. Throughout dinner, she struggled constantly against a compulsion to blurt it out. She succeeded in restraining herself. Then she had the dream, but the event of the preceding day did not occur to her during her analytic hour until the hour was half over.

In this situation are several "levels" of unconsciousness. The deep lack of confidence in me remained still unconscious at the end of the hour and required many subsequent hours for clarification. This deeper level I shall not discuss here. Less deeply repressed but nevertheless with motives outside awareness were the reactions to the interpersonal situations, on the one hand the compulsion to be critical of me to another, and on the other to conceal genuine doubts she had felt the day before from me

The deep lack of confidence laid the basis for a feeling of insecurity with me although at the same time she was dependent. Because the dependency was coupled with distrust there appeared the character pattern of needing to appease me by submissiveness and flattery. This was not conscious to her. Also an attitude of which she was unaware was a tendency to be very critical of me. This further increased her insecurity with me and this increased the need to appease me. The conflict produced the situation where the critical remark made about me was clearly conscious when she was having dinner with another patient of mine, but it was "forgotten" for some time in my presence. This demonstrates the play of interpersonal factors in producing repression. With me, the fear of my retaliation should she criticize me or should I discover she had wanted to belittle me to another, plus the feeling of power at having something "on" me about which I did not know, were potent repressing factors, although they themselves were not entirely conscious. The compulsive nature of her need to tell the friend was produced by at least two trends, the need to tear me down and some genuine desire to be reassured by him. If he had expressed disagreement with the person making the criticism, her anxiety could have been alleviated, but the conflict between her need of reassurance and her destructive attitude towards me was finally rationalized as "I must not tell him because it will shake his confidence also." I say rationalized because she presently documented the fact that the person making the criticism of me was one for whose opinion she had no genuine respect. So somewhere not too far from awareness was the realization that my other patient would probably not be at all devastated by it.

This over-simplified description of a complex situation illustrates the importance of unconscious factors in daily behavior as well as the relative nature of the state of being outside awareness. Repression occurs in and out of daily life in response to situations. There are many popular observations of this. One says, "I am not myself with her," a recognition that some important part of "me" does not seem to be accessible in the presence of a certain person. Reich, Horney and Sullivan have especially written of this. It has been one of the important fields of research since 1925.

It will be said that the present-day study of the manner in which interpersonal forces bring about repression does not invalidate Freud's theory that the reason the ego must develop these defense mechanisms is because of the strength of unconscious instinctual forces which threaten to destroy its relation to the world. As a theory, it has a right to stand until conclusively disproved. But another theory presented from time to time by different analysts should also be thoughtfully considered. Freud's assumption is, in the main, that society is right and the qualities which man must repress in order to get along in society are those which are not good for him.

Jung was the first one to mention the possibility that unconscious aspects of a person were not necessarily undesirable traits, that many potentialities of a person remained unconscious, and that one of the tasks of analysis was to develop these. He felt that thinking people had usually not sufficiently developed their feeling side and feeling people needed their thinking side brought out, etc. Rank, in his conception of the creative artist, also implies that good qualities are often repressed in conforming to society. Fromm has pointed out that the more destructive the culture, the more constructive aspects of the individual may be denied expression, so that one of the causes of suffering and unhappiness is the unlived life.

Sullivan, in his theory of the evolution of the self-system, says that the self-system consists of a person's qualities which have been found to be acceptable to or recognized by the significant people of early childhood and that there is a tendency to dissociate all other aspects of the personality.

Thus, according to him, if the early experiences with significant people are inhibiting, derogatory, rejecting or otherwise destructive, positive aspects of the personality will be forced into "disassociation."

So it is not possible to make a rule about what kind of material must be repressed *per se*. Aspects of the individual tend to be repressed which create too great difficulties in the specific social milieu which is important to the person. Thus in Victorian society a woman had to repress or look askance at her healthy sexual impulses if she was to be accepted.

Psychological processes become or remain unconscious as a result of interpersonal situations. For that reason there is a great variation from time to time and from person to person in the kind of experience or behavior tendency repressed. There are also different degrees of removal from awareness. There is not a sharp line between preconscious and unconscious; there are many borderline situations where merely the fact that an individual is in the presence of a friendly tolerant person or group readily makes awareness of a repressed attitude possible. At the same time, there are many repressions which are very inaccessible. This is especially true of the earliest repressions and character attitudes.

There is much still to be learned about dissociation. A method of research originally used by Breuer and Freud has recently been rediscovered, namely hypnosis. Through it there have been significant findings in two general directions which may further clarify our conceptions of unconscious processes. One is the experiment of "regressing" patients to earlier years of their lives. When this is done there may appear a child of whatever age desired, a one-, three-, seven-year-old and so on, with his emotions and experiences completely unmodified by later life development. It is not yet clear how universal this is nor what it means about unconscious processes.

Another type of research being conducted with hypnosis may eventually shed light on the way irrational attitudes become incorporated in the personality. That is the observation that patients not only carry out post-hypnotic suggestions but that they rationalize the carrying out so that the behavior seems to belong to consciously planned intention. Thus a subject was told that after "waking" from hypnosis he would abruptly leave the room when a certain entirely innocuous remark was made. He responded to the suggestion but said as he left the room, "I must go and see if my car is all right. It just occurred to me that I probably forgot to lock it." By thus explaining his act to himself he does not have to become aware that a thought had been introduced into his mind by another. This tendency to rationalize post-hypnotic behavior was first pointed out by Freud himself.

chapter five

RESISTANCE AND
TRANSFERENCE

Not long after the discovery of free association as a means of bringing repressions into consciousness, difficulties began to appear in the clinical application of the idea. Freud soon discovered that patients could not maintain free association uninterruptedly, that in spite of frequent exhortation sooner or later the patient would fail to mention something which occurred to him. Some of the omissions were due to distress or shame at the thought, and some omissions were rationalized as being too unimportant to mention. Also it frequently happened that patients said *nothing* occurred to them.

In other ways also patients invariably sooner or later showed signs of difficulty with the treatment process. They would come late for appointments, forget appointments or suddenly get involved in acting out their difficulties in life instead of talking about them in analysis. Or they would seem to lose interest in their own problems and turn all their attention to trying to win the love of the analyst or engaging in a competitive battle with him. Freud soon noted that no patient was so single-mindedly serious about his treatment that some one or another of these difficulties did not appear. Since it always happened, he concluded it must be a part of the process and must have a meaning. As early as 1892 he chose the name *resistance* as a general term for this behavior.

He noted further that there seemed to be two types of resistance—conscious and unconscious. Conscious resistance had to do with the conscious withholding of information. This might be associated with some distrust of the analyst or a desire to make a good impression or a fear of rejection. The patient could usually be persuaded to overcome these conscious difficulties.

Unconscious resistance was more significant and more difficult of resolution. In the course of trying to understand this, Freud made the discovery of transference, one of the greatest discoveries in psychiatric therapy. Today both resistance and transference are much more thoroughly understood, but one should never forget the daring courage of Freud's original formulation.

An early conclusion about the cause of unconscious resistance was that it must be produced by the same forces which had, in the first place, created the repression. After an unbearable idea was put out of the mind, according to Freud, there was a constant tendency on the part of this repressed idea to return to consciousness. He thought that the same force which originally repressed it continued to exert a counter-force against its return. It was this counter-force which manifested itself as resistance as soon as an attempt was made to get at the repressed idea. As the situation is understood today, the counter-force is furnished by the defense system of the Ego. Any attempt to break this down produces anxiety, a feeling which the individual always seeks to avoid. So the threat of anxiety furnishes the motive for resistance to insight.

It was soon seen that resistance was not merely a phenomenon which appeared early in the analysis and was eventually completely overcome. Obstruction to progress repeatedly appeared whenever significant data were under discussion. Resistance, in short, was a conservative force seeking to keep the status quo.

One very important source of resistance is what Freud called the secondary gain of illness. By this term he referred to the use a patient could make of his symptoms to manipulate his environment. Thus a chronic invalid might succeed by her suffering in getting attention from a neglectful husband. A person fearing to go alone on the street often manages to demand the constant attendance of a member of the family. More subtly the character trends give secondary satisfaction. Thus an obstinate person may succeed in forcing others to bend to his will, etc. Freud pointed out that this secondary gain was not the primary motive producing the illness but was discovered and utilized only after the illness had developed. At any rate it was believed that the motive of secondary gain alone could not produce neurosis. When it was present, however, the patient had a greater stake in keeping things as they were, and for this reason it furnished a formidable resistance.

Another very significant form of resistance is what Freud termed "acting out." Instead of becoming aware through discussion of the things he does to create difficulties for himself, the patient proceeds to create a difficulty in his characteristic fashion. This can appear in a social or business relationship where it can often do him real damage, or it may (and eventually always does) appear in his relationship to the analyst. It is this last situation which led Freud to his formulation of the concept of transference. He saw this first as chiefly a device utilized to maintain repression. As the name implies, Freud conceived of it as a transferring to the analyst of feelings and thoughts relating to parent figures of an earlier period of life. The analyst, so to speak, takes on the characteristics of these people. The patient than reacts as if he were a small child and the analyst were the father. However, he is unaware of what he is doing. Freud thought that the situation which the patient was re-living in this way was always the situation at the time of the original repression. By re-living it blindly the patient avoided understanding its significance.

If the original problem had been related to incestuous love for the father, for example, instead of remembering it, the patient became absorbed in loving the analyst, and this appeared as an apparent obstacle to cure. However, this behavior, which seemed to be an obstacle, Freud soon realized, could be utilized to bring the patient conviction about his past experience. He could be shown that his feelings were not pertinent to his relation to the analyst but that they must have had meaning at some earlier time. In the experience in the analysis the original situation was merely being re-lived with all its appropriate affect. Transference, therefore, came to be recognized as an important source of insight. By re-experiencing the original situation the patient became convinced of the reality of his earlier experience and was able to see its significance in his life.

Freud soon defined transference more precisely as a repetition of the attitude towards the parents at one particular period in childhood, the period of the Oedipus complex. This was a logical assumption if all neuroses began at that time. So he observed that, with almost monotonous regularity at some stage in every analysis, the patient began apparently to neglect his problem and concern himself with the analyst.

Female patients seemed usually to focus on an erotic interest in him. It did not matter whether they were his age, much younger or much older. All showed a desire to win his love with the belief that if only this could happen they would be cured.

Male patients tended to develop a hostile attitude towards him, to resent his authority and become competitive. Freud saw these two characteristic reactions as part of the Oedipus situation. It was the little girl again trying to win her father's love and the little boy competing with the father for the mother. Consistent with the sexual theory of neurosis, the attitudes were always thought to relate to an erotic situation. Therefore, the definition of transference, which was not modified for many years and in fact is still considered the only true definition of transference by some analysts, was the re-living of the Oedipus situation with the analyst.

Since this characteristic behavior of the patient appeared no matter what the analyst did, it was seen that the transference attitudes did not really apply to the therapist personally. Hence he must not be seduced into thinking the woman had fallen in love with him, nor should he believe that the man hated him. The analyst should rather consider himself a kind of mirror in which the patients' own problems were reflected. According to this early formulation, all attitudes on the part of the patient towards the analyst were considered transference, because there was supposedly no knowledge of and therefore no reaction to the analyst as a person in his own right. In order to facilitate such a situation, the analyst was advised to give no information about himself; to sit behind the patient so that his facial expression was not observed, and to avoid social contact with the patient.

However, Freud recognized that certain things about the analyst could not be concealed. These, he thought, were often used as pegs on which to hang transference attitudes. Thus the actual sex of the analyst was something to which the patient reacted. Some characteristic of personal appearance might serve as an aid in identifying him with someone in the patient's past. In the case of Dora,[1] Freud suspected that his cigar smoking was utilized by the patient in this way. It is now known that there are in addition more subtle ways in which the analyst's personality is involved in the picture; that it is not possible for him completely to conceal the kind of person he is. Thus the patient's attitude is a blending of transference and realistic appraisal.

The patient-analyst situation is, therefore, not as simple as Freud originally thought. Not all attitudes towards the analyst are transference attitudes. One can like or dislike him for what he really is. This means that the total picture is more complex than the mere automatic re-living of a situation from the past with a mirror analyst.

[1] *Collected Papers*, Vol. III, Case 1.

Between 1900 and 1912, Freud's simple formulation of transference was in accordance with his conception of neurotic processes at that time. One was in search of *the* memory or memory complex which produced the symptom and which, when understood, would clear up the patient's problem. One discovered it by transference to the analytic situation of the childhood situation producing it. Today this still is an adequate explanation of some aspects of what goes on in therapy. Such vivid, almost hallucinatory re-living of fragments of the past with complete unconcern for any part of the current reality can be observed from time to time. Sometimes a patient is so overwhelmed by feelings from the past that he distorts even the appearance of the analyst. Brown eyes may become blue. A short-haired analyst may discover she was seen with long curls. One of the most frequent distortions is picturing the analyst as much older than he or she is.

The early description of transference was correct as far as it went, but it did not cover all the irrational attitudes of patients. Much more than the erotic feelings of the Oedipus period is transferred to the analyst, and there are not only other kinds of transferred attitudes than the sexual, but also all kinds of attitudes may come from other periods of life as well as from the Oedipus situation.

The limitations of the early conception were one of the reasons that Freud assumed that some patients were incapable of transference. His assumption that narcissistic people had no libido free to form attachments to other people was based on the fact that most of them did not show the particular Oedipus picture described; they seemed to have no tendency to form an erotic tie to the analyst. This made for a non-therapeutic situation according to Freud's thinking, because if the libido could not move away from the Ego to become attached to the analyst,[1] there was no way of freeing it from its childhood fixation. Thus, the theory led in part to a dead end and until 1912, at least, as previously discussed, psychoanalysis as a method of therapy was believed to be effective only with hysteria, obsessional neurosis and phobias. All other forms of personality disorder such as psychoses and character neuroses were considered not amenable to therapy.

Although this was the official attitude about treatment, even as early as 1911 a few analysts were attempting to analyze "narcissistic" people, and with some success. Also by 1920, analysts were being urged to undergo a personal analysis, not only in order to learn the technique but in order to gain insight into their own personality problems. Since most of these analysts were not supposed to be suffering from neurosis, the only recognized province of analysis, this was a tacit admission that analysis at least had hopes of expanding its scope.

From 1910 on the concept of transference was gradually expanding, but it is difficult to follow the changes since almost nothing was written about it. One is impressed in reviewing the literature with the comparative infrequency of any discussion of the subject which today occupies the central place of interest in theory about therapy.

About 1920, with Freud's formulation of the repetition compulsion, transference again came under scrutiny. Possi-

[1] See discussion of narcissism in Chapter 2.

bly the idea of the repetition compulsion is a crystallization of the development which had been going on. Freud now believed that transference was an outstanding example of the repetition compulsion. The idea of an automatic tendency to repeat earlier life experiences, unpleasant as well as pleasant, gave the concept room for expansion. At about the same time there were again signs of discontent with the existing status of analysis. This time the discontent was about the lack of therapeutic success, and the belief grew that there was a need for a more vital analytic situation. It was thought that the procedure had become too intellectual, and that a more emotional re-living by the patient of his past problems in his analysis would remedy the difficulty. Also the old method of free association did not seem to be very effective with character problems. Whether the discovery of the theory of the repetition compulsion provided impetus for the new developments about the analytic situation cannot be estimated. The fact is that the two things were closely associated in time, and eventually the concept of repetition compulsion was utilized in the new development of character analysis.

By 1927 when Reich had formulated the idea that defensive character trends constituted the chief resistance in analysis, these trends were unobtrusively and without a struggle included under transference phenomena. These were seen as repetitive life patterns. So one no longer thought of transference only as a term applying to libidinous situations of the Oedipus period. Long standing ways of reacting (habitual patterns of behavior), most of them from periods of life earlier than the Oedipus situation, were seen to have

the same irrational quality as the other transference phenomena. Some classical analysts today do not call these attitudes transference but believe the word should be used
only in its original meaning. Many other analysts, however,
do think of them as transference. Sullivan has attempted to
avoid confusion by creating a new term to include the whole
picture, namely *parataxic distortions*. This term, however,
has a rather special meaning, as discussed later. A clear and
specific terminology is obviously important, but it is also
important to see that, in the dynamic processes of the personality, character attitudes perform functions very similar to
transference. Both are reaction patterns taken from the past
and applied indiscriminately to the present situation where
they are not suitable. In the process of making the patient
aware of them as he is acting them out, he is able to see their
role in his difficulties, and this has a therapeutic effect. So
the patient not only tends to re-live childhood situations
with the analyst, but he shows all his customary ways of reacting to people with the analyst.

Not only was the working of character trends in the personality being clarified in the 1920's in Europe, but in the
United States Kempf at about the same time and Sullivan a
little later were demonstrating some therapeutic success with
psychotics by analytic methods. Sullivan's studies in schizophrenia made it clear that the so-called narcissistic people
of Freud are capable of transference, that these people also
transfer to the analyst attitudes and feelings from earlier
stages in their lives. The indifference or distrust so frequently
shown towards the analyst by psychotics is just as truly a repetition of earlier patterns as the hysteric's "love" or competi-

tiveness. In fact, Sullivan and Fromm-Reichmann have demonstrated that the behavior of the psychotic is almost completely transference in the sense of being taken from other frames of reference and having little relation to the analyst in reality. Indeed, one of the difficulties with psychotics is that so much of what they experience is transference phenomena that they find it harder to grasp the real situations than do neurotics.

Another change in the thinking about transference as a result of the formulation of the repetition compulsion is also significant. Before the 1920's, it was assumed that transference occurred according to the pleasure principle. One re-lived an experience in analysis instead of remembering it because one wished to experience again the forbidden satisfaction. This assumption is no longer necessary if transference is seen as an automatic tendency to re-live life patterns, both pleasurable and unpleasurable. This, at least, was a less cumbersome concept, but there was room for further growth.

Reich took a bold step when he showed that character patterns could be used as forms of resistance in analysis, but he still clung to a libido formulation of them. He kept the Freudian theory that character defenses were the result of libidinal sublimations from the pre-Oedipal stages of development. Nevertheless, by his discovery of an active method of interpretation of these to the patient he made an effective modification of psychoanalytic technique. In brief, he found that people with oral characters tended to develop a parasitic clinging to the analyst; people with anal characters were usually stubborn and obstructing, etc. These ways of reacting he repeatedly pointed out to the patients in all situations in which they occurred until the patient became thoroughly conscious of them. He hesitated to call this active interpretation true analysis. Rather he thought of it as a preliminary stage. The character traits were obstacles to be removed, after which one then went on with the analysis, which was the recall of the infantile amnesia. Today no such distinction is made by those who have developed similar techniques. I especially refer here to Horney and Sullivan. With them the analysis of character trends is considered an integral and important part of the development of insight; that is, it is also psychoanalysis.

At about the time Reich was formulating theories about character analysis and Sullivan was working with psychotics, the idea that analysis is an interpersonal process, although not yet specifically called this, was beginning to develop. Sullivan was heading in that direction. Rank vigorously presented his thesis that the analyst must be an active participant and thus definitely become a part of the analytic situation. Ferenczi was noting that the way the analyst felt towards the patient was reacted to by the patient, and that an analyst could not help a patient towards whom he could not feel friendly. Moreover, he noted that many times the patient made correct observations of the analyst's reactions, and he came to the revolutionary conclusion that it would greatly help to develop the patient's sense of reality if the analyst would admit when the patient's reaction to him was not due to his own transference attitudes but to a reaction to the real situation. This new interpretation of the analytic experience is not accepted by all analysts. Many even today maintain that the analyst can and should remain entirely outside the situation, and they especially view with concern the possibility of the analyst's admitting any defects in his behavior. It is feared by them that this would destroy his authority. Those working with the interpersonal concept find, however, that weakening the analyst's irrational authority is part of the process of cure. To the extent that his authority is exaggerated by over-estimation and transference, it must be destroyed. A possibility of some appraisal of the therapist in reality facilitates the clarification, and the resulting relationship is based on genuine respect.

Freud always knew that it was sometimes not possible for the analyst to remain entirely out of the picture, that sometimes, in spite of everything, he would react personally to the patient and what he said or did. This he saw as counter-transference, by which he meant that analysts sometimes transfer elements from their past (or present) problems to the analytic situation. Thus one might be susceptible to the flattery of a patient's erotic interest or one might be hurt by a hostile attack on a vulnerable spot. Because of the stress on the unfortunate aspects of the analyst's involvement, the feeling grew that even a genuine objective feeling of friendliness on his part was to be suspected. As a result, many of Freud's pupils became afraid to be simply human and show the ordinary friendliness and interest a therapist customarily feels for a patient. In many cases, out of fear of showing counter-transference, the attitude of the analyst became stilted and unnatural. Perhaps some of the lack of therapeutic success of the 1920's can be traced to the patient's inability to express his feelings in the cold atmosphere of a stiff, reserved analyst. Rank and Ferenczi were both impressed by the sterile artificiality of the analyst's role at this period. I think it is clear that Freud's conception of counter-transference is to be distinguished from the present-day conception of analysis as an interpersonal process. In the interpersonal situation, the analyst is seen as relating to his patient not only with his distorted affects but with his healthy personality also. That is, the analytic situation is essentially a human relationship in which, while one person is more immediately detached than the other and has less at stake, he is nevertheless an active participant.

By 1929, Sullivan had begun to formulate his theory of interpersonal relations. In this theory, his elaboration of the concept of parataxic distortion is probably the most comprehensive statement of the idea of transference today. In the late 1920's, Sullivan demonstrated that certain psychotics, contrary to Freud's belief, were capable of establishing a relationship to the analyst, and that this relationship showed transference factors, that is, it had irrational aspects growing out of past experiences of the same nature as Freud had found in neurotics. He saw that the gradual clarifiying to the patient of what he is doing to and how he is reacting to the significant other person, the analyst, constituted the process of cure. Out of it a new type of interpersonal situation is eventually integrated. At first glance, Sullivan's observations seem to have much in common with those of Reich about defensive character traits and of Fenichel in his description of habitual attitudes. All three have made observations about character structure.

However, Sullivan's theory of the origin and evolution of the personality differs greatly from that of the classical school, and this also means a different formulation of the development of parataxic distortions from the classical transference picture. Sullivan uses neither the libido concept nor the repetition compulsion as formulated by Freud. Parataxic distortions, according to Sullivan, develop from the early but essentially non-sexual integrations with significant people. One develops ways of coping with these people and then tends to apply these ways in later interpersonal integrations. However, the need to repeat is by no means as rigid a compulsion as Freud formulated in the repetition compulsion. Later experiences can modify the pattern consciously and unconsciously. In fact, the process of cure is an example of such a modification. The analyst, by his objectivity and insight, fails to conform to the patient's expectations and this, when the patient realizes it, constitutes a new interpersonal situation which helps to make clear the irrational nature of his own behavior.

Transference has been much more extensively studied since 1925 than before. The increased interest in the analytic situation with the resulting relative loss of interest in the recall of the past has facilitated this. Out of concentrating on the immediate reactions has developed an understanding of the dynamic function of character structure in obstructing insight.

Besides Sullivan, others of the cultural school have made significant contributions to the theory of transference. Fromm, in his comparing of rational attitudes to authority with irrational attitudes, has demonstrated an important aspect of transference.[1] Janet Rioch, in her paper on trans-

[1] See Chapter 10.

ference, has presented a theory of the way in which transference attitudes are formed.[1] She suggests that the dogmatic commands of parents and their general attitude towards the child, which also is like a command, has an effect similar to a post-hypnotic suggestion. Subsequent obedience takes place blindly, and the parents' evaluation of the child remains to influence and form the basis of the unconscious picture of himself that he carries into adult life.

Some mention should be made of the aspect of transference especially stressed by Horney. She agrees in general with Sullivan's formulation, but she also has another idea which she sometimes seems to emphasize to the exclusion of other aspects of transference. She thinks of the analytic situation itself as producing a special reaction. She sees it as a situation in which there is a struggle for power. This she believes is an essentially new situation in the present, and is a reaction to the overwhelming threat to the neurotic defenses. If we take the example of a female patient in love with a male analyst, Freud would see this as a repetition of the Oedipus situation. Sullivan would see this as a way of reacting to a male in authority, which has a definite history from the past and a present function in relation to the particular male, the analyst. Horney would stress almost exclusively its relevance in the power struggle. It might be a device to disgrace the analyst, make herself feel his equal, "win a scalp," establish a secure position with the analyst without having to change, etc. In short, she sees the transference chiefly in terms of how it is utilized for secondary gain. This makes the interpersonal

[1] *A Study of Interpersonal Relations,* ed. by Patrick Mullahy, Hermitage Press, New York, 1949, pp. 80-97.

situation between analyst and patient essentially a hostile one. The patient envies the analyst's position and resents his advantage over him. So each one tries according to his character pattern to destroy the analyst's power. She does not deny that the patient may have tried similar ways of reacting in other situations, but there seems to be a tendency to minimize the importance of discussing these, especially if they were much earlier or in childhood. However, the secondary gain is certainly one aspect of the interpersonal situation, but should not be stressed to the exclusion or deprecation of others.

It is difficult to discuss transference without becoming involved in discussing therapy. This is a topic in its own right and it therefore seems best to leave further discussion of the therapeutic aspects of transference for a later chapter.

chapter six

THEORIES ABOUT ANXIETY

THE IMPORTANCE OF THE ROLE OF ANXIETY IN the formation of neurosis and neurotic character structure has been discovered only in the last twenty-five years. Prior to the early 1920's, anxiety was considered of little consequence in the development of neurotic disorder. In fact, in Freud's first formulations in 1894 he considered anxiety purely a physiological reaction to the frustration of the sexual orgasm. He believed it did not produce neurosis although he was aware that it was often present in neurotic people. He felt that either there was no significant connection between the anxiety and the neurotic symptoms, or in some cases the neurosis was responsible for a frustrated sexual life and so indirectly was instrumental in producing anxiety. In *The Problem of Anxiety* in 1926 Freud first published his new theory, in which he accorded anxiety a significant position in the development of neurotic disorder. Research in recent years tends to confirm the important premise of Freud's second theory, namely that neurotic behavior is developed in an attempt to cope with anxiety.

In the preceding chapters it has been shown that Freud's

theories about his early discoveries of unconscious activity, repression, resistance and transference have been amplified in the course of the years, but the original thinking remains as a kind of core around which later ideas have developed. The same cannot be said of his theory of anxiety. His second theory of anxiety is not a development or amplification of his first, but a concept at complete variance with the first.

In Freud's first statement about anxiety he placed it entirely outside the realm of neurosis. He believed it was produced as a result of the frustration or incomplete discharge of the sexual orgasm. He thought the blocking of the normal sexual discharge produced a subcortical dissipation of somatic excitation, which was experienced as anxiety; that is, theoretically the physiological-chemical components of sexual tension became transformed into anxiety. No neurotic mechanism was necessary for this and the cure was the practical adjustment of the current sexual life. He was led to this conclusion by the fact that in all cases of anxiety he found a history of sexual abstinence or disturbed orgasm. For example, virgins and young married women who had not yet achieved orgasm during intercourse seemed especially prone to anxiety. It was found also in men practicing coitus interruptus and men living in a state of celibacy, etc.

That anxiety was purely a physiological reaction seemed plausible because often the patient could describe no psychic content accompanying his feelings. He felt anxious but could think of nothing which might be worrying him. Furthermore, in every case of anxiety without exception Freud was able to demonstrate a history of disturbance in the current sexual life, which had resulted in incomplete discharge of sexual tension. He noted, however, that frustration of the orgasm did not always produce anxiety, that some people had a greater tolerance for abstinence than others. This did not strike him as remarkable, for, he pointed out, etiological factors are always more prevalent than diseases in general, and constitutional tendencies and/or the amount of exposure determine a person's susceptibility.

Presently Freud's attention was drawn to the frequency of the appearance of neurotic symptoms in a patient also suffering from anxiety. At first he thought this pointed to a double etiology. In these cases would be found a repression of childhood experiences in addition to a frustrated current sex life. At first he did not think of the two etiological factors as interacting, but eventually he concluded that the presence of inhibitions makes it more likely that a person will be forced into a situation of sexual frustration and therefore he will be more likely to experience anxiety. A psychically healthy person does not endure a state of sexual abstinence indefinitely. If he is not neurotically inhibited, he finds some practical solution.

His early conception of anxiety thus had two stages which may be expressed schematically as follows:

1. *Frustrated sexuality often is physiologically converted into anxiety.*
2. *Sexual inhibition through neurotic difficulties produces sexual frustration, which then becomes physiologically converted into anxiety.*

The second formulation establishes a link between neurosis and anxiety; nevertheless, it is important to remember that although according to this theory the neurosis contributed to producing the anxiety, the anxiety was not seen as due to struggling with the neurotic problem itself but was still thought to be produced as the result of frustration of the orgasm. However, the neurosis appeared first, in contrast to the present-day theories, which are all based on the idea that anxiety causes the neurosis; that is, that the development of neurotic defenses is an attempt to cope with anxiety.

Freud's first theory fitted well into his libido theory. Just as a quantum of energy (or libido) could be bound in a hysterical symptom, it could also be transformed into anxiety. If the orgasm represented the perfect discharge of libido and the end result which the organism was always seeking, it was logical to assume that any disturbance of the process would result in significant changes.

This theory placed anxiety outside the realm of psychoanalytic investigation for many years. However, there is evidence in Freud's writing during these years that he was not entirely satisfied with the formulation, that he felt it left something unexplained. He early noted that anxiety and fear were in some way related emotions. He therefore looked for something in common in their precipitating causes, but with his first theory he could not find a satisfactory connection. He saw clearly that fear was a reaction to danger; in his terminology fear is a part of the Ego's instinct of self-preservation, but he was unable to find a similar explanation for anxiety.

Finally, in 1926, with his new insight, he made the connection and concluded that anxiety was also the signal of danger, a danger from within. Just as fear calls for the defensive measures of either flight or attack, anxiety is a signal for defense. The special types of defense called out by anxiety are symptoms and the character defenses of the Ego.

It would seem that at this point Freud had definitely taken up a new position about the role of anxiety, although he never entirely abandoned his first position. In *The Problem of Anxiety* he struggled to reconcile the two. He speculated that possibly the first reaction of anxiety was due, as he had originally thought, to a transformation of libido but in later experiences the anxiety was merely a signal from the Ego that a similar danger threatened. However, he concluded that it was no longer very important to establish whether anxiety is transformed libido or not.

With this gesture towards the past, beginning in the 1920's Freud's interest in the subject became chiefly centered in the relation of anxiety to symptoms. The first theory offered an explanation of the cause of anxiety. It was the result of the interference with the orgasm either by external events or inhibitions. With the new theory the physiological basis of anxiety remains obscure.

There has been, however, an attempt to formulate a theory of the type of experience which might have first laid the pattern of anxiety in the soma. Rank found the answer in the trauma of birth first proposed by Freud, and the latter was somewhat intrigued by the development of his original idea. The physiological symptoms accompanying the temporary asphyxiation at birth are almost identical with the symptoms accompanying anxiety; i.e., rapid heart beat, difficulty in breathing, and diarrhea. Freud made the suggestion that the birth experience with its overwhelming threat to life could lay down the pattern which then in later life tends to be repeated in situations of danger. But Freud could not concur with Rank's further elaboration of the theory. Rank's idea was that the trauma of birth was especially significant because it dealt with a separation—the separation of the child from the mother—and that all subsequent anxiety-producing situations dealt with threatened separations from something, in weaning separation from the breast, in the threat of castration fear of separation from the penis. Freud criticized Rank's theory on the basis that the child could not know that his danger situation at birth had to do with separation and therefore the idea of separation could not have been a part of the original pattern. He also took exception to Rank's assumption that the child had visual memory-traces from the birth experience.

Even if we assume that the birth experience lays the pattern for all later anxiety, the question must be asked—why some people are more prone to anxiety than others. Since birth is a universal experience of mammals, it was suggested that possibly the predisposition to anxiety was in some way related to the difficulty of labor. Folklore seemed to lend some support to this—for example, "Macduff was from his mother's womb untimely ript" and so without fear, referring to a Caesarian birth.[1] There has been very little attempt to study the relationship between difficult labor and anxiety. Greenacre[2] suggests that more than the actual birth process must be concerned in the formation of the original pattern

[1] Macbeth, Act V, Scene VIII.
[2] Greenacre, "The Predisposition to Anxiety," *The Psychoanalytic Quarterly*, Vol. X, 1941, pp. 66-94.

of anxiety, that experimental observations on foetal activity prove the existence even at that time of anxiety-like patterns. She concludes that constitution, prenatal experience, birth and the situation immediately after birth all play a part in creating the predisposition to anxiety. One can speculate that disturbing emotions or organic disease in the mother may by direct chemical transmission sufficiently alter the soma of the foetus so that he remains permanently more susceptible to disturbing experiences. However, this is still very much in the realm of speculation and although it is an interesting field of research it does not greatly concern the practical therapist at the present time. The fact is that the reason why some people develop anxiety more readily than others is still unknown. It cannot yet be determined whether it is due to some congenital predisposition or whether certain types of early life experiences lay the foundation for the predisposition. The problem in fact seems to be but one aspect of a more comprehensive question. What makes some people more sensitive, more deeply affected by life experiences than others?

There is a need to know rather what anxiety is about and how the organism copes with it. This is the field in which most research on the subject in recent years has been done. As it was pointed out earlier, Freud's second theory of anxiety, published in 1926, started constructive thinking on new angles as to the significance of anxiety. He at last established to his satisfaction that anxiety is about the same kind of thing that fear is—that it is a reaction to danger. Just as fear is a reaction to known, chiefly external danger, anxiety is a reaction to unknown danger from within oneself. This, he believed, gave anxiety its peculiar character. One cannot run away from it nor fight it by the methods used to cope with fear because the danger is a part of oneself. Some people deal with the danger by projecting it, that is, making it appear to be external danger, as in the phobias where the patient complains not of distress about inner difficulties but fear of cats, snakes, high places and so on. Or it may be dealt with by repression and the erection of defenses against its return to consciousness. Both projection and repression tend to conceal the true nature of the danger and to mobilize the forces of the personality against a substitute. As a result the general feeling produced is one of helplessness. One does not know what the danger is or where it is. The situation is similar to that of someone hearing a noise in a dark room. Since nothing can be perceived, the imagination can concoct weird dangers, thoughts which are quickly dispelled when a light is brought and the noise is found to be produced by something commonplace such as a shade flapping in the wind.

Freud described the anxiety-producing situation as follows. Some force or forces within the person threaten his relation to the outside world. The dangerous forces within arise from two sources—the strength of the instincts and the severity of the Superego. The strength of the instincts threatens to overwhelm and force the Ego to commit acts unacceptable to the outside world. This threatens the Ego in various ways at different stages of development. In the earliest years it threatens the immature personality with loss of love. This danger Freud sees as catastrophic because it means to the helpless infant loss of the mother who feeds and protects. At a later stage the breaking through of forbidden instincts exposes the child to the threat of castration, and still later forbidden behavior brings the disapproval of society which produces the fear of ostracism. The severity of the Superego is related to the last-mentioned dread. Because of it the child fears not just the reality-disapproval of society, but attitudes of society which he has incorporated within himself. This "conscience" contains much that is irrational and harsher than the real demands of society. So in time anxiety is produced by the struggle within the person of the harsh Superego and the powerful forbidden instincts.

Freud's theory assumes that the forces within the Id are of dangerous proportions, the danger being greater or less according to the relative strength of the Ego. The earliest experiences of anxiety occur when the Ego is still weak because it is in the process of developing. This early experience sets the pattern for all later life. Having been dangerously threatened once, the Ego tends to assume that the same situation will always be a danger to it. So in later life when similar situations arise, anxiety appears as a warning. This is a signal for the defenses of the Ego to go into action. In the meantime the Ego has actually become stronger but it is not free to notice this, for the signal of anxiety acts automatically and the Ego, assuming it is again threatened with annihilation as it was originally, meets the danger according to the old pattern. That is, the body again automatically prepares itself by its various physiological mechanisms for flight or attack. One might say that anxiety acts like an air raid alarm. There are false alarms and times when the danger does not require the use of all defensive measures, but each alarm nevertheless calls out the full defensive resourcefulness of the city (the Ego).

So where the particular dangers experienced in early childhood are concerned the Ego continues to act through life as if it were as helpless as in childhood, and anxiety originally a response to real danger becomes merely a signal that such supposed danger again threatens.

Freud's conception forms the foundation for more recent work on anxiety. That impulses and drives within a person often threaten his relation to his fellow man is a generally accepted thesis today. That the possible outcome of this is loss of love, ostracism, and even the possibility of being deprived of a part of himself (not necessarily just his penis) also seems to state the situation accurately. There is, however, a difference of opinion about the nature of the impulses within, and pertinent new observations have been made.

Freud's theory that man struggles throughout life to cope with powerful innate fixed impulses is consistent with his theory of the nature of man, a theory at variance with the observations of modern anthropologists and social psychologists. The differences will be discussed at greater length in the next chapter. Briefly, Freud sees man as possessed of two powerful drives, the life (chiefly libido) drive and the death instinct. These man must struggle to control throughout life in order to maintain a secure position in society. The danger of losing control of these impulses produces anxiety.

Culturally oriented analysts today agree that anxiety appears when something within the person threatens his relation to significant people. However, the inner impulses which threaten security are now seen to be largely forces created by cultural pressures. There are innate drives, but they are not anxiety-provoking. Most of the dangerous pressures are created by rage and hostility in reaction to frustration. The innate instincts of sex and aggression considered so powerful by Freud are not believed by these analysts to be of overwhelming strength in themselves. Rather, the formidable force within is generated by the repression of the resentment and hostility created through the frustration of one's potentialities, "instinctual" and otherwise, by the pressures of the society in which one lives. This constitutes an ever increasing force within pressing towards outward expression which would bring loss of love and approval.

In recent years contributions to the theory of anxiety have been made by three analysts: Fromm, Horney and Sullivan. Since there has been much exchange of opinion and free discussion among these three, each one's contribution is in a way the result of the joint research, and the various points of view do not contradict but rather supplement each other.

All three disagree with Freud as to the nature of the threat from within which produces anxiety; that is, all three are of the opinion that the threat from within is produced by cultural pressures.

Of the three, Sullivan has described in the greatest detail what may be called the basic anxiety or the earliest pattern of anxiety. He sees the need of approval from the significant adult or adults as the essential atmosphere for the growth of the young human organism. When the atmosphere of approval is present, the child has a feeling of well-being, called by Sullivan *euphoria*. Disapproval is immediately felt as loss of euphoria. This is a state of discomfort which becomes eventually known to the child as anxiety. Very early the child begins to make efforts to avoid the feeling of anxiety, and the self of the child is formed as a result of this effort. In other words, the child tries to make himself behave always in a way which brings only approval or the sense of euphoria. The parents help the child to learn many things, some of which one might call rational in that they represent part of the equipment necessary for survival and mastery of life, such as learning to walk, learning to distinguish real dangers such as fire, etc. Education in these things is not anxiety-producing, or at least need not generate lasting anxiety patterns of pathogenic power. The parents also educate the child in more irrational things; that is, in certain inadequate or contradictory aspects of the mores of the particular culture in which he finds himself. Here it is harder for the child to see the sense or practical usefulness of some of what he is taught. He learns it solely for the sake of maintaining the feeling of euphoria, that is, for the sake of avoiding disapproval and escaping anxiety. For this reason he acquires many of the social graces, toilet habits, table manners and thousands of subtler ways of feeling and acting which go to make up the behavior of an acceptable citizen of a particular culture. For example, in our culture one attitude confusing to the child is that it is all right to play with one's fingers and very bad to play with one's penis. It is, according to Sullivan, the process of exposure to the cultural pattern that produces especially significant anxiety situations.

Fromm's view, which does not disagree with Sullivan's, expresses it differently. He sees the early pattern of anxiety growing out of the conflict of the need for closeness and approval and the need for independence. Sullivan and Fromm both show that in the need for the approval of the significant adult the trends which the growing child tends to curb in himself *are not necessarily undesirable traits per se.* They are merely trends which are at variance with the approved cultural norms. Fromm especially stresses that some of a person's best potentialities may meet with the disapproval of a destructive parent, or may be sacrificed because they do not conform to the norm of a particular culture. Under such circumstances any attempt to express positive potentialities may produce anxiety. Thus a culture in which cruelty is considered evidence of strength and power tends to repress in its people all expression of kindliness and impulses to help the weak. To take an example from our own culture, we may consider a child of middle-class parents to whom making money has become a symbol of success. Suppose the child early shows marked artistic talent. The father had planned another career for his son—perhaps in business—perhaps in a profession. He views with dismay his child's budding talent. If he is an extremely dictatorial man, he may do something pretty definite to put a stop to this "nonsense." If he is a man who consciously feels he should not interfere with his child's development, he may suffer in silence. But, even so, the child soon gets the feeling that this creation of his for some reason does not please. One of three things may happen. He may become defiant about it and struggle ahead; he may become secretive and paint or draw only when his father is not around; or he may accept his father's decision and conclude painting is a "bad" thing to do. In the third case he decides presently that "there is no money in it," that it is almost impossible to become famous at it anyway, and so on. All three are possible ways of coping with the anxiety produced by his father's disapproval. It will be noted that the father's displeasure was not about a destructive trait in the child but about a positive potentiality. In the attempt to cope with the father's attitude some of the boy's free creativity is lost; in fact, in the third outcome the child becomes completely inhibited about expressing his artistic talent.

The pattern for producing basic anxiety described by Fromm and Sullivan has something in common with Freud's theory in that all agree that impulses within the child threaten his relation to others to the extent that he may lose love, be punished or be ostracized.[1] Horney's views of the basic anxiety are not as extensively elaborated as Sullivan's and Fromm's. She stresses a little more that the frustrating situation tends to make the child hostile, this in turn leading him to feel that the world is hostile, and this belief increases his sense of helplessness.

A great difference between Freud and the cultural school lies in the conception of secondary anxiety. This, as I have shown, is, according to Freud, merely a signal that an old danger threatens. It is still the same danger, i.e., the power of an instinct. The Ego has merely learned by experience how to prevent its erupting before damage can be done. Sullivan and Horney have shown that something much more complicated happens. According to them, the danger producing secondary anxiety is from a new source within the per-

---

[1] I have interpreted the threat of castration here as a general symbol of punishment.

sonality. The situation threatened by it is still the same, the individual's relation to his environment, but they both find that the defense system itself has become a potential source of anxiety.

According to Sullivan's theory, secondary anxiety appears after the self-system is established and all trends in the individual not conforming to it tend to be dissociated. Whenever there is a possibility that the dissociated thoughts or feelings will become conscious, the self-system is threatened and anxiety appears. The dissociated impulses need not be destructive nor likely to produce unfavorable consequences in reality. The fact that recognition of them would change to some extent the nature of the self-system is all that is needed to produce anxiety. In short, by the time the self-system is formed, there is an emotional stake in maintaining it blindly and this forms a rigidity in the personality and increases the potentiality for anxiety.

Horney's theory about the secondary anxiety amounts to something very similar. According to her, the secondary anxiety grows out of the very defenses originally erected against anxiety. A vicious circle is formed in which anxiety produces defenses, which provoke new anxiety, which in turn causes the formation of new defenses and so on. Defenses can produce two types of situations which are provocative of new anxiety. Having a defense or symptom increases one's vulnerability. As was stated in discussing Sullivan's views, the maintaining of a defense system becomes an added responsibility. The person now not only has to adjust to other people and their attitudes, he has to adjust to them without in any way disturbing his defense system.

This makes relationships with others much more dangerous and inflexible. Supposing, for example, a man always has to give the impression of being well informed. This trait was developed at some time to cope with a feeling of inferiority. In order to maintain the pose he sometimes says he has read books he has never opened. As long as no special pressure is put upon him all goes well, but some day a situation may arise in which his ignorance is exposed. Then he either becomes more humiliated and anxious than he would have been had he made no pretense, or he quickly thinks up a new escape or rationalization. So the defense itself can create more anxiety by actually placing the person in a more vulnerable position.

Neurotic defenses can increase anxiety in another way, according to Horney: they may be in conflict with each other. For example, early influences may lead a child to develop a great need of success and recognition. Later contacts may develop in him a contempt for such needs. So he remains secretly ambitious, but with a need to be modest and inconspicuous. Both trends were originally developed in response to a need of approval. There are three general possibilities of personality development as an outcome of the conflicting trends. The person may be so successful that his real worth brings him recognition in spite of his excessive modesty. If this is the case no new anxiety is produced.

It is more likely, however, that the inability to assert himself leads to his talents' failing to receive recognition. This is intolerable to his ambitious side; either anxiety must appear or a new system of defenses is added such as the presumption that he has enemies blocking his progress. Conversely, his ambition may force him to try to break his inconspicuous pose, in which case again anxiety appears or a new defense is formed. These are the people who often collapse under success and readily retreat to a dependent relationship to an authority.

The pyramiding of defenses, each defense coping with anxiety, but in turn laying the ground for new anxiety, constitutes the danger from within, according to Horney.

All analysts, including Freud, agree that repressed hostility is a frequent source of anxiety. Freud sees this as the result of biological forces, a part of the death instinct directed against others. The more recent cultural approach sees repressed hostility as a reaction to frustration or hostility from others. The assumption is that we are born with a tendency to develop and grow. If in the process of growth we meet with disapproval and our interpersonal security is threatened, the rage at frustration has to be repressed because rage also is not tolerated, and the seeds of a dangerous hostility begin to develop. This growing repressed hostility makes us more likely to arouse counter-hostility in others, and this in turn steps up our own hostility and so on. This dynamic interaction, and not an innate instinct, constitutes the dangerous, anxiety-producing force from within.

It is probable that some frustration of the developing personality is inevitable in any prolonged interpersonal situation, but some cultures are more frustrating than others and some parents have a greater emotional stake in moulding the lives of their children than others. The over-protective mother, for instance, greatly increases the child's conflict. She makes the price of security for the child a more or less complete surrender of his independence. This creates frustration and resentment in the child and this in turn threatens his security, and the threat to his security in turn makes him more resentful. The more he fears, the more hostile he becomes; and the more hostile he becomes, the more he fears.

Since 1923 the investigation of anxiety has made significant progress. Freud pointed out the direction by showing that symptoms are formed in an attempt to cope with anxiety. Although he persisted in his idea that the danger within is from the strength of the instincts, he correctly stated the fact that anxiety is produced when the impulses within the person endanger his relation to his fellow man. The ways in which the neurotic character structure itself contributes to the formation of new sources of anxiety was not described by Freud and is a new contribution in recent years.

Research on the problem of anxiety has made progress in answering two questions, namely, what is endangered and what is the source of the danger?

It is seen that any threat to a satisfactory relationship with one's fellow man can produce anxiety, and also any threat to the expression of one's potentialities is anxiety provoking. In addition secondary anxiety is produced by any threat to one's illusions, which are sometimes difficult to differentiate from one's potentialities. The need to be related to one's fellow man and at the same time express oneself may produce a conflict. In order to gain a measure of security in some situations it may be necessary to partially sacrifice the one or the other.

The sources of the danger, therefore, are the irrational pressures of society first felt through the attitudes of the parents, and finally the accumulated difficulties within produced in the process of conforming to the irrational pressures of society.

Anxiety is always characterized by a feeling of helplessness, a disjunctive force. This is due to the fact that the danger is within, and its nature is not known since the original threat was dealt with by repression or projection, and further the anxiety often rises out of a conflict of defense systems, which cannot be resolved by simple means.

chapter seven

FREUD'S CULTURAL ORIEN-
TATION COMPARED WITH
MODERN IDEAS OF CULTURE

SINCE FREUD HIMSELF STRESSED SO MUCH THE
importance of the innate instinctual life in neurotic problems, the fact that he also considered cultural pressure significant may easily be overlooked. Throughout his writings
we find evidence, usually not greatly stressed, of his recognition of cultural factors. The difference between Freud's theoretical orientation and that of the present-day "cultural
school" is not simply that Freud's approach stressed the biological factors. It is also important that Freud's theories
about culture were quite different from those of modern
anthropologists. Freud not only emphasized the biological
more than the cultural, but he also developed a cultural
theory of his own based on his biological theory.

There were two obstacles in the way of understanding the
importance of the cultural phenomena he saw and recorded.
He was too deeply involved in developing his biological
theories to give much thought to other aspects of the data
he collected. Thus he was interested chiefly in applying to
human society his theory of instincts. Starting with the as-

sumption of a death instinct, for example, he then developed an explanation of the cultural phenomena he observed in terms of the death instinct.

Since he did not have the perspective to be gained from knowledge of comparative cultures, he could not evaluate cultural processes as such. As has been stated elsewhere, much which Freud believed to be biological has been shown by modern research to be a reaction to a certain type of culture and not characteristic of universal human nature. Although a genius, Freud was in many respects limited by the thinking of his time, as even a genius must be.

He firmly believed in the authority of the patriarchal family. In the early years of his work, that is, in the period before 1900, he could be critical of parents, or at least of parent substitutes such as uncles, etc. He listened to and for a time believed patients' stories of childhood sex traumata at the hands of adults. But when he found that some of these stories were fabrications, he returned to the conventional attitude that parents were all-wise, loved their children, and could not create problems for them. Thus he could say in the "History of an Infantile Neurosis," [1] in spite of plenty of evidence in that particular case history to the contrary, that ". . . The life of a child under school age is easily observable, and we can examine it to see whether any 'problems' are to be found in it capable of determining the causation of a neurosis. But we find *nothing but* [2] instinctual trends which the child cannot satisfy and which it is not old enough to master. . . ." In other words, if a child is hostile to his father,

[1] *Collected Papers*, Vol. III, p. 528.
[2] Italics mine.

this is due to the child's difficulties. The fact that the father may provoke hostility by his behavior is not deemed important. This was the characteristic attitude of the time.

Also Freud never became free from the Victorian attitude towards women. He accepted as an inevitable part of the fate of being a woman the limitation of outlook and life of the Victorian era. The attitude of the male towards the female of that period was either one of gallantry or brutality. It was the rare person who could treat a member of the opposite sex as a simple human being. We find this reflected in Freud's writing. His chivalrous, and at the same time condescending, statements about women sound strange in a scientific treatise. The castration complex and penis envy concepts, two of the most basic ideas in his whole thinking, are postulated on the assumption that women are biologically inferior to men. This also was one of the fundamental assumptions of the Victorian era. He realized that the limits imposed on women by the culture had something to do with their feeling of inferiority, but he never questioned the origin of the attitude in the culture. He assumed that the cultural attitude was determined by the biological situation.

Another cultural handicap for Freud was his own traces of the Victorian attitude towards sex. The man who first brought the unhealthiness of the current sexual attitude of his era to the attention of his world was himself to some extent the victim of it. In spite of his courageous scientific discussions, there are frequent evidences that he struggled with his own feeling that he was dealing with a "dirty" subject, that he was discussing the baser nature of man, a side of him to be controlled if possible, sublimated, and to some extent regretted. The sexual act itself as a part of creative productive love is a concept not found in his writings. Nowhere is there any intimation that sex can be the expression of the best in human relationships. Sex, according to Freud, is chiefly important as a relief from tension. One does not get much indication of its being part of an interpersonal experience.

To him it is biological that a child should develop shame about his interest in his excreta or genitals. To be sure, he says this development of loathing and shame is *aided* by education, thus paying lip service to a cultural force, but he does not question the correctness of the educational attitude. Such training is assumed to be a part of a necessary indoctrination into knowledge of the facts of life. And so it was in the society in which he lived.

Throughout his writings are to be found references to cultural pressures, but they are never accorded primary importance. For example, basically he thought of the Oedipus complex as an inevitable biological stage of development. At the same time he makes reference to the fact that the mother often prefers her male child, and that the father's attitude towards the little girl may be different from that towards his son. He recognizes that these facts also influence the Oedipus complex. But he considers this biological and natural. Always he recognizes that culture plays a part, but he thinks of culture as the servant of biology. Thus he failed to observe that the neurotic father and mother are more likely to have incestuous attachments to their children than are more normal parents, and that the incestuous attitudes of parents greatly foster the incestuous attitudes in children. In short, Freud assumed that the people he observed were typical specimens

of universal human nature, and therefore the puritanical attitudes of Victorian society were believed to characterize
human nature in general.

Freud's theory of culture was influenced by the limitations
of his personal outlook as well as by his biological bias;
nevertheless, it was an ingenious explanation of the facts
which he observed. It at least recognized that man lived in a
society and was modified by it. His theory was first presented
in 1913 in *Totem and Taboo.* In 1915 a short paper entitled
"Thoughts for the Times on War and Death" showed his increasing interest in the broader cultural implications of his
theories. In the 1920's he turned more definitely to the application of psychoanalytic theory to society and wrote *Group
Psychology and the Analysis of the Ego, The Future of an
Illusion,* and finally *Civilization and Its Discontents.* In all
of them he develops a theory of society consistent with his
instinct theories. It is disappointing to find that Freud took
little interest in the study of comparative cultures which was
coming more into the center of attention in the 1920's. Although he lived until 1939, there is no evidence that his
thinking was in any way modified by the findings of modern
anthropology. Indeed he summarily rejected anthropological
findings which would contradict his theories.[1]

Freud's cultural orientation differs from these findings in
two important respects. The first difference has already been
extensively discussed in this book—namely that much which
is known today to be culturally determined behavior in man
was believed by him to be the expression of unalterable bio-

[1] Sigmund Freud, *Moses and Monotheism,* Alfred A. Knopf, New York,
1939, pp. 206-207.

logical trends. In other words, his concept of man differs definitely from that held by modern anthropologists.

Freud's concept of society was also at variance with recent theories. He conceived of society as a static force, developed as a mechanism for controlling man's instincts. The only change which seemed to take place was that in the course of the centuries it had probably become increasingly a better controlling organization. Because of this belief Freud foresaw man becoming increasingly more frustrated as he became more civilized. Since man was a biological organism striving to live according to the pleasure principle and seeking to give unbridled rein to his instincts, he must inevitably clash with society, the inhibiting force. The two chief instincts in man frustrated by society were sex and aggression. According to his first theory sex was the most important problematical drive, but later he believed man suffered fully as much from the repression of his destructiveness. On several occasions he refers to civilization as having been achieved at the price of the renunciation of instinctual satisfactions.[1] This in brief was his conception of society. All that is cooperative in man, all that is creative, is purchased at the price of renouncing instinctual satisfactions. Man, therefore, must always be restless under the demands of society because his most fundamental urges are being repressed.

In 1913 in *Totem and Taboo* Freud first presented his theory of man's emergence from his animal past. His theory was developed from several sources: anthropological material available at the time (chiefly Frazer); his interpretation of

---

[1] See "Thoughts for the Times on War and Death" in *Collected Papers*, Vol. IV, Ch. 17; also *Civilization and Its Discontents*.

data gleaned from patients; Robertson Smith's totem theory; and conjectures of Darwin's that the first human society must have been composed of a group or groups dominated by a powerful despotic male.

This male, postulated by Darwin, Freud sees as the father of the primal horde. He subjected all the younger males to his absolute power and kept all the women for himself. The sons thus were forced to live in abstinence and in complete obedience until one day, having banded together, they revolted, killed and ate the father. The totem feast is thought to be the symbolical repetition and commemoration of the original criminal act. Presently the sons were seized with guilt and a need to atone. The guilt was a result of the tender feelings for the father. Behind the hate was love. This led to proscribing the killing of the totem and to the deification of the father as the totem animal of the tribe, an animal whose life was sacred except at special feast occasions when he was sacrificed and the ancient crime was symbolically relived. But also the brothers feared each other. The danger was that there would be competition among them to see who would take the father's place and repeat the subjugation of the rest. Hence they renounced the "fruits of their deed" by denying themselves the liberated women. A taboo against killing within the tribe was established. To prevent any male from attempting to seize all the women in the tribe the incest taboo came into existence. By making it compulsory to marry outside the tribe the competition for women was no longer a serious threat to the new social organization.

This was Freud's conjecture about the beginning of human society. It is apparent from the above data that he believed society was created out of the necessity to curb man's destructiveness and sexual drive. It assumes that rivalry, jealousy and lust for power dominate human nature. Modern research in cultural anthropology has not confirmed Freud's theory.

It is important to consider these matters in the history of psychoanalysis because it shows very clearly Freud's conception of the role of society. A group which could work together was finally formed by setting up protective taboos against the so-called natural instincts of incest and murder. This presents man as hostile to his culture and conforming only out of fear. Culture is a kind of rigid police system imposed upon him.

When Freud applied his theory to the society in which he lived he could only express pessimism for the future of man. In *Civilization and Its Discontents* he applies the idea of the original struggle between man and society to modern times. He says that when the inhibiting influences of civilization are removed, we see "men as savage beasts to whom the thought of sparing their own kind is alien." [1]

According to him, man is "good" only because of his helplessness and dependence on others. The attitude of the group towards the individual determines the ideas of good and bad; an act is "bad" if it threatens man's security within his group. This is certainly the attitude which is prevalent in our society. It leaves out of consideration entirely the possibility that some things may be bad for man even though they are socially approved, and that some things socially disapproved may be good, and it implies that there are no socially con-

[1] *Civilization and Its Discontents*, p. 86.

structive tendencies unless the police force, society, insists upon them. In *Civilization and Its Discontents,* society, according to Freud, establishes its hold on the individual through the sense of guilt. The sense of guilt has its origin in the fear of rejection and punishment. Originally the fear related to the parents, but with the incorporation of the parent images within the personality in the formation of the Superego (a part of which is conscience) the sense of guilt serves man's own tendency to punish himself. Freud's theory is that the higher the culture the greater the sense of guilt. The more man renounces, the more guilty he feels about everything. Freud explains this in a rather complicated manner. As long as man only feared external punishment, he could feel safe if his behavior conformed, but when he developed conscience (Supergo) "nothing is hidden from . . . [it], not even thoughts" [1] and they are often "bad" in spite of every effort to control them. So the more man strove to be upright, the more his thoughts bothered him and the more guilty he felt. This he explained also in libido terms. The more a man controls his sadism, the more it increases. It is not permitted to be cruel towards others and therefore must turn the same energy on the self. This attack on the Ego he believed was made by the Superego which had acquired the frustrated aggressive energy of the Id. So the more blameless a man's life is, the more cruel his Superego will be and the more guilty he feels.

Since it was assumed that the pursuit of the pleasure principle meant the unbridled expression of sex and aggression, man's pursuit of happiness was not compatible with unity

[1] *Civilization and Its Discontents,* p. 108.

with his fellow men. So man the individual must always be hostile to society.

Since society makes man increasingly unhappy, he has found various ways of enduring it. For a few very superior souls sublimation is the answer. These people are actually able to diminish the pressure of the instincts by converting them into socially acceptable behavior. Substitute gratifications comfort some. Drinking and smoking are examples.

One great source of comfort for the masses is religion, which Freud sees as a kind of group psychosis, an escape from reality by believing in the illusion of a kind, loving, heavenly father who promises happiness in heaven for those who make the necessary renunciations of their instincts on earth. Freud seems to be thinking chiefly of Christianity here. Some Oriental religions do not fit his description.

Love may also be a solution, but Freud sees this possibility as precarious since it is fraught with the danger of loss of the love object.

Those who do not find one of these solutions become neurotic and thus obtain distorted gratification of the instincts through symptoms. Society on the whole is tolerant of this and may even treat the sufferer kindly without recognizing that its rules are being violated.

War, according to Freud, is the inevitable accompaniment of civilization. Man's aggression is so strongly frustrated and repressed that periodically all of the above palliative measures fail to cope with the inner pressure, and a period of general unleashing of man's animal nature must appear, wear itself out, and peace is once more restored.

This is a brief summary of Freud's theory of the relation of man to culture. It assumes that all cultures are similar to our own, and that the function of society is to curb the biological instincts. These, it is assumed, are dangerously powerful and a threat to human relations. Man's biological tendency to destructiveness is believed to be so powerful that society can only cope with it by periodic wars. Aggression, competition and lust for power are considered basic human drives.

Were we dealing with the realm of pure theory, one could say that Freud's speculation about the development of society and its relation to man at least offers an explanation of most of the facts of this culture. If we did not know that less destructive and more destructive cultures exist, it might be accepted as a valid theory. Modern anthropology has cast doubt on some of Freud's assumptions, such as the universal necessity of war, the universality of the Oedipus complex, the assumption that woman is of necessity the underprivileged sex, etc.

Cultural anthropology is still in its infancy. There is as yet no study of man in other cultures which compares in depth or detail with Freud's psychoanalytical studies of the man of middle-class society in Western European culture.

However, there is adequate evidence that man does not universally conform to the picture described by Freud, and that the variations in his character are related to the variations in his culture. For example, we have found that in one culture where the men greatly outnumber the women, the social position of woman is greatly enhanced and she occupies a position of power.[1] In non-competitive societies war is less likely to occur; in matriarchal society the picture of the Oedipus complex is greatly altered. On the other hand, there are societies where not only is hostility to the outsider fostered but general distrust of each other within the group is taken as a matter of course. There at least is evidence that more than one pattern of human relations can exist. The facts also indicate that society is not just an inhibiting force, but that different societies create different needs and interests in their people.

It seems apparent that the two basic drives, sex and aggression, postulated by Freud are not in themselves problems. Sex is not the same kind of a problem in a culture which does not inhibit it or degrade it as it is a problem in our society. Self-assertion becomes destructiveness only under certain circumstances. Competitive cultures seem to produce a great deal of destructiveness in their people, and non-competitive societies do not. It follows that the universal need of war as a means of coping with man's drives is to be questioned.

The conclusion from the study of comparative cultures is, therefore, that man is not biologically endowed with dangerous fixed animal drives and that the only function of society is to control these. Society is not something contrasted to man but something at the same time created by man and creating man. That is, society is not a static set of laws instituted in the past at the time of the murder of the primal father, but is rather a growing, changing, developing network of inter-

[1] Abram Kardiner, *The Individual and His Society*, Columbia University Press, New York, 1939; see Linton's chapter on the Marquesans.

personal experiences and behavior. One of its functions, Freud correctly observed, is to control social behavior. But it has other functions. In fact it creates man. One cannot become a human being except through cultural experience. Society creates new needs in people. Some of the new needs lead in a constructive direction and stimulate further development. Of such a nature are the ideas of justice, equality and cooperation. Some of the new needs lead in a destructive direction and are not good for man. Wholesale competitiveness and the ruthless exploitation of the helpless are examples of destructive products of culture. When the destructive elements predominate, we have a situation which fosters war.

There seem to be cultures which encourage man's development, and cultures which are predominantly destructive of man's best interests. The latter produce a whole society of psychically crippled and unproductive people. The Kwakiutl and the Dobu described by Ruth Benedict [1] are outstanding examples of the latter. There were and are sufficient destructive forces in the Western culture to have made the development of the fascist character a reality.

Outstanding among those who in recent years have made a study of the relation of man to his society is Fromm. Trained in the social sciences as well as in psychoanalysis, he retains a broad social perspective in studying psychological phenomena. He is alert to economic and political factors in society, and thus is in a position to make certain new suggestions about the relation of man's problems to cultural pressures.

[1] Ruth Benedict, *Patterns of Culture*, Houghton, Mifflin Co., New York, 1934.

"Freud," he points out, "accepted the traditional belief in a basic dichotomy between man and society, as well as the traditional doctrine of the evilness of human nature. Man, to him, is fundamentally antisocial. Society must domesticate him, must allow some direct satisfaction of biological—and hence ineradicable—drives; but for the most part society must refine and adroitly check man's basic impulses. In consequence of this suppression of natural impulses by society something miraculous happens: the suppressed drives turn into strivings that are culturally valuable and thus become the human basis for culture. . . . The relation of the individual to society in Freud's theory is essentially a static one: the individual remains virtually the same and becomes changed only in so far as society exercises greater pressure on his natural drives (and thus enforces more sublimation) or allows more satisfaction (and thus sacrifices culture)." [1]

Freud, in effect, Fromm maintains, enshrined those passions and anxieties characteristic of modern man in Western society as fixed biological drives.

For Fromm, "those drives which make for the *differences* in men's characters, like love and hatred, the lust for power and the yearning for submission, the enjoyment of sensuous pleasure and the fear of it, are all products of the social process." [2] Although human beings have certain common needs, like hunger and sex—and even these are not fixed as to form of expression and fulfillment—man's nature, his passions and anxieties, his thoughts and acts are a cultural product.

---

[1] Erich Fromm, *Escape from Freedom*, Farrar & Rinehart, New York, 1941, pp. 10-11.

[2] *Escape from Freedom*, p. 12.

Man moulds history as well as being moulded by history. While his energies are organized and channeled by the process of acculturation, they at the same time become potent forces, either constructive or destructive, depending on circumstances of history and locale and family, in further moulding of the social process. Human nature thus has certain characteristic dynamisms and laws which react back to alter man's situation. Man is not static; he is a dynamic entity which changes the course of history while being changed by it. A product of historical evolution, he is both carrier and creator of history.

One can express this more concretely by saying that man has not only imperative physiological needs but an equally imperative need to be significantly related to the world and to himself in order to avoid intolerable loneliness and isolation. If he is to preserve his sanity, man must have some kind of spiritual relatedness to the world, some frame of orientation and devotion, whether he finds it in organized religion or in some secular institution or in a comprehensive idea.

Fromm approaches the problem of human relatedness from two sides, the one phylogenetic, the other ontogenetic. From the phylogenetic aspect, man has emerged from the relatively fixed instinctive adaptation of his animal ancestors. This, of course, was a long-drawn-out process, but it has resulted in a lack of inherited specific action patterns. This obliges man, in the most literal sense, to learn how to live. At birth he is completely dependent on others. Gradually he learns how to walk, eat, etc., without help, how to communicate, how to cooperate with others and to get along in society. Since he has no inherited fixed courses of action, he has to learn how to act, and since there are competing possibilities of action, he has to think. Thus man gradually learns to look upon himself as an entity separate from the rest of nature and from his group. He becomes aware of his powerlessness in the face of the cosmic setting. And he becomes aware of death as his ultimate fate though he may disguise it or deny it in numerous phantasies and rituals.

In this way man has gained freedom from more or less blind and instinctive adaptation to nature, where there is no organized consciousness and no thought of the morrow, no awful feeling of isolation and no thought of death. But man's self-awareness remained dim for long periods. Through his participation in a clan, or a social or religious community, he gained a feeling of security and belonging. He was no longer tied to the natural world like an animal, but he was tied to the social world he was born into, his group. Thus his need to be related to the world in order to escape his powerlessness and feeling of isolation was solved, or rather did not develop. He had a determined place in relation to his group, which implicitly defined what he was and how he should live, and which gave him security.

But such a tie, as long as it obtained, blocked further growth, for it circumvented the need or necessity for developing his critical capacities, his reason and imagination beyond a certain point. But here again man's fate overtook him. He could not remain tied to his group. Reason and imagination, through a variety of historical circumstances, disrupted his unquestioning relation to his group and to his world, which had defined his fate. He became aware of the incompatibilities of his existence, of the brevity of his life.

Self-consciousness intervened. He began to think about death, injustice, human exploitation.

Thus human development is said to have a "dialectic" character, forever posing a dilemma of opposing situations. On the one hand, man becomes more free in that his reason and imagination, in fact all his powers, over a long period develop more and more, resulting in greater mastery over nature and the vicissitudes of the material world. But reason and imagination as they grow remind him more and more of his precarious situation, of his isolation, of his inevitable end, of all the incongruities of human life. And thus he cannot rest. Once man has set out on the road which leads away from animal existence and from unselfconscious social participation, he cannot return to his original state. He cannot escape the contradictions he finds in life—he must face them. He must reconcile himself to death and his situation in a cosmos indifferent to his fate. He must also recognize the problems created by his society, problems which can in time be modified by his contribution.

Fromm chooses the Western European culture as a specific example by which to develop and illustrate his thesis. Since this is a culture which, since the Middle Ages, has been in process of rapid change, it demonstrates especially clearly that neither man nor his society are static in relation to each other. The influence of social forces in abolishing former values and creating new needs can be easily observed in the swiftly changing picture.

Through the Middle Ages, man in the Western culture was a part of a structuralized whole with a definite role in his society. His life had a definite meaning, but he had no freedom of choice. He was the role he played in society and identical with it, a peasant, an artisan, a knight. His individual personality did not count, did, in fact, scarcely exist. At this time awareness of oneself and of others as separate and unique persons had not yet fully developed.

The new economic, political, religious and social movements which followed the disintegration of medieval life changed all that. A powerful moneyed class, for example, rose during the Renaissance, filled with the spirit of initiative, power and ambition, ruthless and indifferent to the claims of human dignity. The masses became a "shapeless mass" who were to be manipulated and exploited. Wealthy nobles and burghers used every means at their disposal, including physical torture, to rule over the masses and check their own competitors. The security of a stable long-standing social structure was destroyed and man had to seek a new role.

The result of all this, and much more, was an increasing sense of helplessness, isolation and insecurity. Men were more free in that their status no longer was tied to their place in the social order; birth and origin counted less. Individual initiative for those who were in a position to exercise it counted for more. But men were more alone; they no longer belonged to a meaningful moral and social totality. "All human relationships were poisoned by this fierce life-and-death struggle for the maintenance of power and wealth. Solidarity with one's fellow men—or at least with the members of one's own class—was replaced by a cynical detached attitude; other individuals were looked upon as 'objects' to be used and manipulated, or they were ruthlessly destroyed if it suited one's own ends. The individual was absorbed by a passionate egocentricity, an insatiable greed for power and wealth. As a result of all this the successful individual's relation to his own self was poisoned too. His own self became as much an object of manipulation to him as other persons had become." [1]

The new freedom brought both an increased feeling of strength born of successful economic activity and wealth and an increased isolation due to the life and death struggle, resulting in anxiety. During the Middle Ages a social and moral order existed which gave man's life meaning. Now doubt and skepticism arose as to the meaning and significance of life.

It is not necessary for the purpose of this book to discuss Fromm's account of the Reformation and the rise of Protestantism. The two opposing tendencies mentioned above—growing freedom and growing isolation—were strengthened. In different social classes the new-found freedom of course differed in quality and degree. The wealthy capitalist could enjoy more of the fruits of the new freedom. The position of the middle class was more insecure; its freedom brought more isolation and personal insignificance and less of confidence and strength. Burning resentment against the powerful and rich upper class was strong. The lower classes, who had little to lose and much to gain, were impelled by a new quest for freedom and an ardent hope to end oppression.

Protestantism, says Fromm, not only gave expression to the feelings of the average member of the middle class. It increased and strengthened them. It taught him to despise and distrust himself and others.

[1] *Escape from Freedom*, p. 48.

Omitting many details, I want to mention the fact that, in Fromm's explanation, a new type of character emerged. The individual developed a readiness to submit to the purposes of an extra-personal power. By complete submission to the divine power he could be loved by God and hope for salva· tion. Success became a mark of divine favor, and hence a compulsion to work and to save developed. Such traits be-came productive forces in capitalistic society. At the same time they allayed anxiety and doubt and gave the individual some personal satisfaction.

Hence on the one hand modern man learned to rely on himself and on his own effort, to make responsible decisions. Capitalism freed him from social and political shackles, as did Protestantism from spiritual shackles. He became in·creasingly free from the bondage of nature. Knowledge grew. These factors, among others, contributed toward the de-velopment of an active, critical responsible self.

At the same time he became more alone and isolated. Everything depended on his own efforts and luck. He was no longer a part of a corporate order. He was alone. Protestant · ism did not allow him to face God as an integral part of a group through the intermediary of the Church. He had to face God alone too. Everywhere he faced superior power, God, competitors, impersonal economic forces.

Essentially, in Fromm's view, modern man is characterized by these two sets of opposing traits. Certain more recent trends have, in fact, exaggerated them. The question is whether he will be able to maintain his self-reliance and in-dependence while he finds some solution to his feeling of aloneness, or whether he will give up his integrity and freedom in order to feel once again related to others at no matter what loss of freedom. This is a hazardous course, for man cannot reunite himself with the world in the way he was related before the development of individuality. The price to be paid is a stunting of personality and often compulsive activity. Thus no real happiness can be found in this way, and his problems remain, unconsciously if not consciously, to bedevil him. All neurotic phenomena are examples of this attempt at "solution." The ways in which man tries to escape from the problem of individuality are by Fromm labeled mechanisms of escape, which I have elsewhere discussed.

We have thus two concepts of the relation of man to society—Freud's and that of the cultural school. Freud's outlook is completely pessimistic. From his point of view society, by its very nature, forces man to repress his inborn aggression more and more. The outlook for the future is that the more civilized he becomes, the more potentially destructive he becomes.

The view that man's destructiveness is largely a product of social pressures, while painting no rosy picture of the present state of civilized man, at least does not lead to a theoretical dead end and a needlessly stultifying pessimistic conclusion. One is justified in assuming that not all the forces at work in a changing culture are proceeding in the direction of more and more inhibition. It is theoretically possible that new constructive forces may be introduced; that favorable changes in the culture will react favorably on man, and that comparable changes in man will react favorably on the culture.

Freud's fatalism is reflected in his therapy. With his point of view, the best that can be done for a man is to make him more able to accept the restrictions of society. With the new point of view the goal of therapy is different. The aim of the "cultural school" goes beyond merely enabling man to submit to the restrictions of his society; in so far as it is possible it seeks to free him from its irrational demands and make him more able to develop his potentialities and to assume leadership in building a more constructive society.

chapter eight

DEVIANTS AROUND 1912.
ADLER AND JUNG

In the first chapter i pointed out that at three points in the development of analysis significant changes in outlook have occurred. The first change occurred around 1900 in Freud's own thinking with the diminishing of his interest in the theory of the traumatic origin of neurosis, and increased concentration on innate tendencies as producing neurotic developments.

The second period of transition began around 1910 and had to do with a growing feeling that the sexual theory of the neuroses was either unsatisfactory or at least incomplete. As has been shown in Chapter 2, Freud himself eventually added aggression as an important non-libidinal factor in neurosis. Before Freud reached this conclusion, however, two of his pupils had made more revolutionary attacks on the theory that sexual libido was the stuff of which neurosis was made. These two were Adler and Jung. Both of these men had significant modifications to offer, but unfortunately, fairly early in their course of disagreement, both were separated from the group around Freud. Thus the main stream of analysis was deprived of what might have been fruitful controversy eventuating in an early integration of the positive contributions of the two men with Freud's contribution. It would seem too that because of the isolation there was a tendency on the part of Adler and Jung to over-emphasize differences, and this in general often results in exaggeration of the importance of the controversial points.

Both Adler and Jung attacked the libido theory, each in a different way, but in so doing each made new contributions. In fact, although some of the observations made long ago by them were rejected by classical analysis for many years, these have eventually become accepted in some form, usually without acknowledging the priority of the formulations by Adler and Jung. Thus, for example, Freud's discovery of the importance of aggression was anticipated by Adler, and later attempts to deal therapeutically with ego defenses at many points echo Adler's approach. Jung's contribution is less tangible, but he was the first person to bring up for consideration the importance of the interaction of analyst and analysand as well as of parent and child, and he was the first person to state that positive aspects of the individual could be repressed.

ADLER

Adler was the first pupil of Freud to be severed from the psychoanalytic group. His departure in 1911 was the result of the tension developing around his rejection of the sexual etiology of neurosis. It will be seen in subsequent chapters that this is usually the moot point whenever a serious schism resulting in actual separation has occurred. The strictly biological instinctual emphasis of Freud's outlook seems to have been the one issue on which he could not tolerate questioning. For him the validity of psychoanalysis stood or fell by the libido premise. In discussing the deviations of Adler and Jung he concludes, "What is left over [omitted], however, and rejected as false, is precisely what is new in psychoanalysis and peculiar to it" [1]—that is, the importance of infantile sexuality (libido and the instincts).

Adler saw inferiority feelings as universal in human beings. He first developed this idea in connection with organ inferiority, which might be morphological or functional. It seemed that a person tended to do one of two things with organ inferiorities. In the first case he substituted another organ for the inferior one. An example would be developing strong arm muscles to do some of the work of partially paralyzed legs. Or he concentrated on the inferior organ and strove to overcome its inadequacy as the stutterer, Demosthenes, according to tradition, became a great orator. Adler noted that the body itself tended without conscious volition to compensate for weaknesses. Thus the diseased heart hypertrophies in order to carry on its function. These observations about organic inferiorities produced no controversy with Freud.

Presently, however, Adler enlarged his thinking on the matter. He observed there was also a tendency to compensate in the psychic life for organic inferiorities. The mind seemed to center on the inferior organ and try to find some way of feeling superior about it. This, he saw, tended to lead into a world of phantasy unless one did actually have some success in becoming superior. Thus a little girl who heard her mother

[1] *Collected Papers*, Vol. III, p. 527.

lamenting about her (the little girl's) plainness might build a phantasy of being a beautiful princess sought after and loved by everyone. This, of course, could not solve her problem in reality.

Adler enlarged his theory still further. The existence of an inferior organ was not required. He thought that a child by the very fact that he is small and helpless feels inferior, and that therefore there is a universal feeling of inferiority in humans. In addition to this certain attitudes on the part of the parents favor the development of feelings of inferiority. Among the attitudes mentioned are lack of tenderness, neglect, ridicule.

Out of the feeling of inferiority grows the need to enlarge one's ego feeling by dominating or finding a way of feeling superior. This Adler saw as the need to be "the complete man," which he called a "guiding fiction," a kind of neurotic goal. The striving for superiority need not necessarily end in neurosis. A man may actually become successful because of his attempts to overcome inferiority feelings. However, many compensations embody ideas and goals far removed from practical possibility. In these circumstances the goals become distinctly neurotic.

Adler saw the male as the symbol of power in Western society. Therefore strivings for power could be called masculine. Woman was in an inferior position; thus the term feminine could be used as a symbol of inferiority. So there is a tendency on the part of all to acquire a more masculine ideal and strive for that. To this striving Adler gave the name "masculine protest." The masculine protest is characterized by a drive to get from the "below" position to the "above" position. It is especially marked in women, but it is found in all people in weak positions. He even saw flight into illness as a way of getting power. Such a person dominates by helplessness and often succeeds in forcing others to make compromises in adjusting to his illness. Adler implies that this may be the primary motive for illness instead of one of the secondary gains as Freud and most others see it.

Instead of sex the search for power determines man's actions and development. Here is Adler's major clash with Freud's thinking. He differed also on another point which did not seem to disturb Freud as much as the rejection of the sexual. He saw Freud's approach to neurosis as one of seeking the initial causes; the emphasis was on the past. His own approach placed the emphasis on the future. He emphasized the purposive nature of human behavior. One becomes neurotic in the pursuit of "fictive goals."

Adler not only discarded the idea that sexual drives were at the root of neurosis but he went to the opposite extreme and said that in the person seeking to feel superior the sexual act is also involved and is *nothing but* a struggle of two people to have power over each other. The Oedipus complex also, according to him, is the attempt of the boy child to subjugate the mother and fight successfully with the father. When the Oedipus complex persists into maturity, it is because the child has been pampered and so is timid about reaching out into life. The erotic attachment then becomes a device for clinging to the parents for security.

According to Adler there are two general ways of dealing with inferiority feelings. There is the flight into illness, where one gains a feeling of superiority from getting attention and from manipulating the environment; secondly, the need to compensate is expressed in a more open struggle for power. In the course of trying to become the "complete man" one sometimes achieves considerable success in terms of recognized achievement.

Thus around 1910 Adler presented an entirely new theory of neurosis, which discarded many of the essential points of Freud's thinking. For the sexual drive he substitutes the will to power as the guiding force in human behavior. Also in placing all the emphasis on the pursuit of goals, he minimizes the importance of any understanding of the initial cause. There is an oversimplification of the picture which gives the impression of superficiality and led Freud to feel that Adler denied the existence of the unconscious. The unconscious as understood in 1910 did not include the unconscious defensive activities of the Ego later described by Freud and subsequently studied extensively by Reich, Anna Freud and recent workers. So in the terminology of the time Adler had turned his attention away from what was considered the true province of psychoanalysis, the unconscious instinctual life, but he had discovered a new area of research, to be investigated more than ten years later by Freud himself, namely the unconscious defensive function of the Ego. To be sure, Adler in 1910 did not see this clearly, but all unwittingly he had formulated the beginnings of a method of character analysis—he had shown that use of neurotic conditions for power or satisfaction purposes is also an unconscious process. What he described very effectively was the situation of man in a competitive culture. He stated very clearly that woman's inferiority feelings had to do with her position in the society

in which she was living. He observed also that woman, as
mother, was the transmitter of the culture to the child. The
fact that in the course of struggling with his difficulties man
seeks to solve his problems by the search for the way to feel
superior and thus actually often further complicates his difficulties was also an important discovery. It has much in common with Horney's "Idealized Image" and Sullivan's idea
that maintaining an inadequate self-system is a potential
source for increasing anxiety. I think not even Freud would
deny the truth of many of Adler's concepts. His criticism was
this: "From a highly composite unit one part of the operative
factors is singled out and proclaimed as the truth; and for the
sake of this one part the other part, as well as the whole, is
repudiated. If we look a little closer, to which group of factors it is that has been given the preference, we shall find that
it is the one that contains what is already known from other
sources . . ." [1] This statement was made apropos the thinking
of both Adler and Jung.

Adler's description of the possible power uses of sexual
activity could conceivably have thrown light on Freud's puz-
zle about compulsive heterosexuality and promiscuity. It will
be recalled that Freud felt at a loss to explain them as neurotic manifestations because since libido is being discharged
in these conditions, there should, according to his theory, be
no neurosis. Adler was the first one to point out that sexual
disturbance, instead of causing neurosis, was but one of the
situations where neurosis manifested itself. However, Adler
overemphasized the role of the struggle for power in the sexual life. Although in our culture competitiveness is generally

[1] *Collected Papers*, Vol. III, pp. 526-527.

pervasive and is rarely totally absent from the sexual relation, nevertheless he overlooked the existence of non-competitive love.

Freud made another criticism about Adler which, in view of the subsequent development of psychoanalysis, can clearly be seen as "dated." In 1914 he wrote: "Psychoanalysis has never claimed to provide a complete theory of human mentality as a whole, but only expected . . . to supplement and correct the knowledge acquired by other means. Now Alfred Adler's theory goes far beyond this point; it seeks at one stroke to explain the behavior and character of human beings as well as the neurotic and psychotic manifestations. It is actually more suited to any other field than that of neurosis." [1]

One can criticize Adler's views on some of the same points as Freud did. He did attempt to build a whole system on the basis of a partial view; he oversimplified the problem of neurosis and at least in one of his earliest writings, *The Neurotic Constitution,* he did not make entirely clear how much of the behavior he was talking about is unconscious. However, according to some pupils who worked with him in later years, he did not deny the existence of the unconscious as that term is used today.

But Adler's positive contributions to psychoanalysis are significant and, as I have already pointed out, he anticipated by several years a more general acceptance of several similar ideas. He was a pioneer in applying psychoanalysis to the total personality. He was the first to observe that much which was at that time called constitution is itself to a great extent

[1] *Collected Papers,* Vol. I, p. 338.

the product of attempts at adaptation. Indeed "at one stroke" he enlarged the field of psychoanalytic exploration. He was the first person to describe a part of the role of the Ego in producing neurosis and to show that the direction in which a person is going, that is, his goals, significantly contribute to his neurotic difficulties. The unfortunate thing here is that he tended to substitute his idea for the causal approach whereas, as Jung long ago observed, it seems clear that both are significant and that the pursuit of neurotic goals develops after the first damage to the personality is done. Another important contribution of Adler's has been his awareness of cultural factors. He came to see that a woman's feeling of inferiority, for instance, is related to her underprivileged position in society. And finally he was the first person to discard the sexual theory of neurosis.

Adler eventually established his own school of thought and called it Individual Psychology. In his treatment he greatly modified the therapeutic procedure taught by Freud. There was an active attack on the patient's overt difficulties. Short treatment was the rule and Adler himself considered his method of a didactic nature, that is, a form of re-education. His great practical contribution in recent years lay in his advice about the parent-child situation.

JUNG

The next pupil to break with the Freudian thinking was Jung. Jung had a different background from that of Freud and most of his pupils. He had a more extensive experience with psychotics and he had a wide knowledge of the myths, symbolism, literature, and philosophy of many cultures. From all of these sources he had rich contributions to make to psychoanalysis and these were at first welcomed. Jung never fully accepted Freud's sexual theory, but for many years there was no open quarrel about it. Rather, Jung's observations developed side by side with Freud's. In his thinking he did not utilize the sexual theory, but at the same time he did not openly contradict it. As early as 1909 Jung concluded that the neurotic difficulties of parents were the decisive influences in the difficulties of children. He said, "What most influences him [the developing child] is the peculiarly affective state which is totally unknown to his parents and educators. The concealed discord between the parents, the secret worry, the repressed hidden wishes, all these produce in the individual a certain affective state which slowly but surely, though unconsciously, works its way into the child's mind, producing therein the same conditions and hence the same reactions to external stimuli. . . . If grown up persons are so sensitive to such surrounding influences we certainly ought to expect more of this in the child whose mind is as soft and plastic as wax. . . . The more sensitive and mouldable the child the deeper is the impression." [1] Thus Jung early observed the subtle interaction of child and parent, a factor in the development of neurosis too much neglected by Freud.

He also early brought more sharply into the foreground a consideration of the importance of the mother, thus emphasizing an influence in the child's life earlier than the Oedipus complex. Because of his emphasis on the mother, Jung stressed regression as an important neurotic craving, being in the last

[1] Carl Jung, "The Association Method," *The American Journal of Psychology,* Vol. XXI, No. 2, April, 1910, pp. 246-247.

analysis the desire to return to the mother and finally the womb as a symbol of security or rebirth.

There are several other aspects of Jung's thinking which, while not like Freud's, did not definitely repudiate Freud's ideas. For example, Jung gave a more extensive interpretation of symbols than Freud. Freud saw symbols as usually reducible to a sexual meaning. He thought of them as representations of psycho-sexual activity. Jung felt that this did not cover all cases of symbolism, that the symbol also had a forward-moving significance, that sexual symbolism can be saying something about the future, about a positive purpose in life. So he points out that instead of concluding that all symbolism has a sexual meaning, sex itself is sometimes used as a symbol of something else.

Jung's real split with Freud came in 1912 when, among other things, Jung presented a new interpretation of the libido. In his reformulation as it appeared in *The Psychology of the Unconscious,* he suggested that the sexual libido was only one form of the "primal" libido. This primal libido he finally defined as synonymous with undifferentiated energy. He referred to it as psychical energy and gave it the general meaning of a life force. He did not deny that a great part of this libido could be conceived as originally sexual in character, but it had become desexualized and could no longer be reconverted into sexual energy. So although he makes a revolutionary denial of the sexual origin of libido, he seems to define it in almost the same terms as Freud. He does something similar with the Oedipus complex. He sees it as a symbol of childhood ties to the parents which must be broken in the emancipation required at puberty, but he also apparently sees it as Freud does as a stage in development having erotic features. However, there is no doubt that Jung (and Freud) considered his thinking a departure from Freud's. Certainly he definitely maintained that obtaining pleasure is not necessarily identical with gaining sexual satisfaction.

Jung did not deny the importance of early childhood in producing neurosis. As I have pointed out, he definitely saw that the tensions of parents had to do with moulding the character of the child, but he denied that sexuality was an important factor in early childhood. Jung denies that the activities of the child prior to the period which Freud called the Oedipus period should be considered sexual. He sees this period as related to growth and nutrition. There is a hint at this point that he would like to make nutrition the origin of all other drives. For example, he compares the rhythmic machinery of sex with sucking. Whatever interest there is in the genitals he sees as a naïve investigating. He describes the mother as the first love object but the interest in her is not sexual—she is rather the food-providing, nourishing being. In other words, translated into Freud's terminology, the first attachment of the child has to do with self-preservation, not sex.

Jung sees sexuality as beginning to be a factor in the later years of childhood—pre-puberty—and then from puberty onwards, he grants sex a very important role. Thus clearly Jung's picture of the origin of neurosis and the relative importance of various early childhood experiences is quite different from Freud's. There is a lack of stress on the biological and sexual, while the reaction of parental tensions on the child's developing personality is given great importance.

Jung makes another related observation out of which developed an aspect of his thinking for which there would be no room in Freud's theory. This is the idea of the repression of positive aspects of the personality as well as forbidden instincts. He saw education as producing a conflict. He saw it as confining a person and diverting him from his "individual line" of life. The meeting of this conflict and the search for self-realization (individuation) became an important part of his later system of therapy.

Jung differed from Freud in the goal of therapy. Freud's method he described as causal, giving a retrospective understanding. A functional analysis looks to the future and strives to find the meaning in the present and future. In his own method he would combine these two aspects. In practical terms he questioned whether recalling the past and explaining the present situation in terms of the past were adequate. He felt there must be some constructive planning of the future in addition. The combination of the two aims in analysis has been utilized by present-day analysts, although not in the same way as Jung used it. From the need for constructive development for the future, much of Jung's later system has evolved.

Another contribution of Jung's was partially utilized by Freud. This was the idea of the collective unconscious. According to this theory the significant memories of the human race are a part of everyone's heritage. This, Jung thought, might account for the similarity of symbols and myths found in widely separated areas over the earth. Not only the human heritage but also residues from the animal past are a part of the collective unconscious. Freud never definitely stated a conviction about this, but in his theory of the evolution of society from the primal horde he utilizes a similar concept. The taboo against incest, for instance, is believed to be the result of a kind of racial memory of the primal experiences.

Jung utilized his concept of the collective unconscious quite differently. For him it represented the wisdom of the ages. Thus he felt that the collective unconscious contained tendencies superior to the individual's. This had a significant influence on his therapeutic approach. A part of the process of self-development consisted in bringing a person into contact with his collective unconscious. This was done to a great extent through the interpretation of dreams. Jung saw the dream as having meanings on several levels. There was the personal meaning relating to the immediate life of the patient. If one pushed associations beyond that, one finally reached the collective unconscious meaning. Thus a dream about the father would finally come to a conception of all fatherhood, the father archetype. At this level supposedly the knowledge acquired by mankind through the centuries becomes available to the patient. In the search for the meaning of dreams the analyst's free associations were utilized as well as those of the patient.

The participation of the analyst in interpreting the patient's dreams emphasizes another observation of Jung's. According to Jacobi,[1] Jung saw analysis as a mutual process in which the analyst participated. He believed the patient could not progress beyond the point the analyst had reached, but he also believed the analyst could continue to grow through

---

[1] Jolan Jacobi, *The Psychology of Jung*, Yale University Press, New Haven, 1943, p. 66.

contact with his patients. Questions must be raised about the way in which Jung utilized this idea, but the idea itself is very important since it is the first time analysis was seen as an interpersonal process.

After Jung's break with Freud, he turned his attention more in the direction of what he would have called the constructive aspects of therapy, that is, guiding the patient to avail himself of his unconscious wisdom. In the course of developing ideas along this line, his thinking becomes more mystical and he creates a conception of the personality which sounds like a rigid obsessional system. According to his idea there is a male and female side to everyone. If the male is dominant, the female is repressed. The well-rounded individual needs the development of both aspects. Also there are four main characteristics in everyone: thinking, feeling, sensation and intuition. These constitute pairs of opposites. The opposite pole to thinking is feeling, and sensation is countered by intuition. In men, thinking and sensation are usually the conscious characteristics and feeling and intuition are repressed. In women feeling and intuition are uppermost. The repressed feminine side of man is called his *anima*, the repressed masculine side of woman is her *animus*. The task of therapy is to bring these forces into equilibrium; that is, to develop the anima and animus to make the well-rounded individual. This seems to be a fanciful idea. Jung had a theory of character types, already mentioned (Chapter 3), in which these divisions of the personality are utilized. The two main types of character are the extravert and the introvert. Both of these types are dominated by one of the four characteristics. Thus there may be a feeling introvert or extravert, etc.

As the Jungian school has developed, the process of cure has tended to become rigid and ritualized, and patients are said to go through various stages until they finally reach self-realization. One cannot achieve this until after middle life. The system as it stands today has the quality of a religion. Jung believed that people needed a religious attitude, by which he seems to mean a respect for the dignity of human life, and a belief that it has meaning.[1] There is a quality of respect for the patient in Jung's thinking too often not indicated in other analytic approaches.

One other concept of Jung's should be mentioned because it suggests one of the ways in which man conforms to a cultural pattern. This is the Persona (the Latin word for mask). Jung thought that the individual in the course of his life tends to put on like a mask the attitude which is expected of him. Each profession, for example, has its characteristic attitude which the individual tends to wear. The doctor has his Persona, the business man another one, etc. The Persona was considered not a part of the true character although firmly attached to it and not easily removed. It rather acts as a sort of protection of the inner person.

It is not within the scope of this book to make an extensive critical study of Jung's complete system as it has finally developed. Some of his contributions should be considered because of their positive value for psychoanalytic therapy. I also wish to point out the significant negative aspects.

The chief over-all criticism of Jung's thinking is that it

---

[1] Carl Jung, *Two Essays on Analytical Psychology*, Dodd, Mead & Co., New York, 1928, p. 186. ". . . all religious conversions, that cannot be traced to direct suggestion and contagious example, are based upon independent inner processes, the course of which culminates in a change of personality."

tends to take the patient away from reality and substitute a mystical, semi-religious phantasy life.[1] It can be especially dangerous to psychotics in that it encourages absorption in phantasy processes, and therefore strengthens the tendency to confuse reality with autistic thinking. Jung's method of interpretation of dreams is an example of his theory in action. The patient starts with his problem but presently through his associations reaches contemplation of the universal. In contemplating the experience of the race he supposedly finds insight into his own difficulty. This is especially well documented in the analysis of the dreams presented in his book *Psychology and Religion*. One cannot help thinking that in spite of the interpretations the patient's problem still remains but thinking about something else has been substituted for it. This is the classical mechanism of the obsessional neurosis. Another unfortunate aspect of Jung's method is the indoctrination of the patient. If the analyst contributes his associations to the patient's dreams and he starts with a theory about collective unconscious imagery, the end result will usually be indoctrination of the patient with the analyst's theory. It has been said, and possibly with some truth, that Freudian analysts indoctrinate their patients with the sexual orientation, and to some extent any analyst's thinking must have some influence on the patient, but at least other systems do not as actively undertake indoctrination as the Jungian method does.

Nevertheless, especially in his early years, Jung has made positive contributions to the understanding of personality and to therapy. He was the first person to point out the im-

[1] My collaborator, Patrick Mullahy, does not agree with this.

portance of the subtly working neurotic tensions of parents on their children. Although environmental factors were not denied by the Freudian school, they were not studied to any extent, and nowhere in Freud do we find any indication of the importance of the unconsciously working tensions of people on each other as described by Jung. Also Jung was the first person to see analysis as the interaction of analyst and patient. His observation that the analyst's difficulties block the patient's progress and his awareness that the analyst can learn about himself from the patient were new ideas.

Jung had a new concept of what is repressed in man and this meant a new concept of the goal of therapy. Freud felt man had to repress his unacceptable aspects. Jung saw that man also repressed some of his positive potentialities, and he believed that one of the functions of therapy was to bring out the undeveloped aspects of the patient's personality. "Only what is really oneself has the power to heal." [1] Although Jung's idea of what constitutes undeveloped aspects differs greatly from that of Fromm, out of this thinking came a very significant attitude, for which Jung deserves great credit—an attitude of respect for the patient and his neurosis. [2]

The two early deviants from Freud were poles apart both temperamentally and in their approach to the understanding of neurosis. The thinking of each differed from that of the other fully as much as it differed from Freud's orientation. Although they withdrew from Freud's group at about the same time, it apparently never occurred to either to join

---

[1] *Two Essays on Analytical Psychology*, p. 178.
[2] See comparison of "individualism" and "individuation," *Two Essays on Analytical Psychology*, p. 184.

forces. Each went his own way, deviating ever farther and farther from Freud's thinking and from each other's. Yet these two men had at least three points in common. Both were dissatisfied with the libido hypothesis and sought to build a theory of neurosis on a different basis. Both were dissatisfied with the causal therapy of Freud and believed the patient's aims must be considered. Jung saw the understanding of goals as at least as important as the understanding of cause. In Adler's case, he wished to substitute the goal for cause as the all important factor in neurosis. However, the nature of the goals described by the two men is quite different, as the above presentation demonstrates. The third point on which they had much in common was their emphasis on the importance of the child-parent relationship. Jung early pointed out its significance; Adler came to a consideration of children and parents later when Jung had apparently lost interest in the subject. One may note with some surprise that Jung with his background of knowledge of many cultures was not the one to make the most significant observations of the effect of cultural pressures on the individual. Adler was the pioneer in this work. As has been said, the thinking of these two deviants made little impression on the main stream of psychoanalytic thinking for many years. In recent years some of their ideas have been re-discovered. Horney seems to have especially fallen heir to Adler's thinking, while some of the contributions of Rank and Fromm are related to the best ideas in Jung.

chapter nine

DEVIATIONS AND NEW
DEVELOPMENTS IN THE 1920'S

AFTER ADLER AND JUNG WITHDREW FROM THE "psychoanalytic movement," there followed several years in which Freud and his remaining followers continued to think along the lines of the earlier theories. Freud's contributions during this time were for the most part of a highly academic nature. To his theoretical speculations about the unconscious, instincts, narcissism, etc., he gave the name metapsychology. His other writings were in the field of applied psychoanalysis. There were numerous such attempts during this time to apply psychoanalytic principles in a theoretical way to literature, art and various other subjects. World War I for several years required the services of many analysts, thus temporarily turning their attention from their specialty. It was a period of growing pessimism about the therapeutic effectiveness of psychoanalysis. The methods of treatment then in use, chiefly the recall of childhood experience through free association, were seen to be often without therapeutic value. Freud himself had become most pessimistic by 1920. He still felt that analysis had much to contribute in theoretical understanding of human personality, but human nature had proved more unchangeable and intractable than he had supposed.

Yet out of the thinking of this period several brilliant changes in theory crystallized around 1920. Freud presented a new instinct theory, bringing out the importance of aggression and the repetition compulsion. There followed his theory of the total personality, i.e., Ego, Superego and Id, and finally his new evaluation of anxiety. But these changes in theory at first seemed to have little relation to the technique of therapy for several years. Psychoanalysis as a method of therapy seemed to have reached a dead end. Freud himself turned his attention away from the study of the individual and became interested in the study of cultural phenomena.

The need obviously was for some improvement in therapeutic technique, and by 1925 innovations and experiments aiming to increase therapeutic effectiveness were under way. Three names especially stand out: Rank, Ferenczi and Reich. All three eventually met with the serious disapproval of Freud, but for different reasons. Only Rank ended by questioning the libido theory and substituting for it a new theory of personality. Reich, far from questioning it, has given it a central place in his own system. Ferenczi took the middle road. In his earlier years he was a most ardent supporter of Freud's theory. Doubts of its validity gradually crept in; he became more interested in what went on between parent and child and analyst and patient. To the end he kept Freud's terminology but gradually shifted his emphasis to what is now called the interpersonal process.

Therapeutic effectiveness was the goal, and all three in different ways attempted to develop the analytic situation into a vitally effective emotional experience.

RANK

Rank was the first of the three to offer radical changes in therapy, but these changes were closely tied up with a new theory of personality. Prior to the search for an effective therapy, Rank had shown some deviation from Freud. It was within the framework of the biological orientation that he first took issue with him. Instead of according the Oedipus complex the central place in the causation of neurosis, he presented the theory that all neurotic difficulty stems from the trauma of birth. Freud had earlier pointed out that certain physiological accompaniments of the birth process (especially difficult births) were also found in anxiety states. Rank did not stop at this. He found the psychological situation of birth very significant. On both the physiological and psychological levels he saw birth as a profound shock. This he believed produced the primal anxiety which constituted a kind of reservoir of anxiety within the person which was slowly dissipated in the course of a lifetime. Portions of it are released in all later anxiety-producing situations. The physiological and psychological aspects of the birth situation had to do with the trauma of separation from the mother. Rank thought that all later experiences involving a separation acquired a traumatic quality because of the first trauma. This is what makes weaning, separation from the breast, and the threat of castration, separation from the penis, foci for anxiety. Thus all anxiety can be interpreted in terms of birth anxiety. Freud pointed out that awareness of being separated from the mother at birth could not possibly exist, nor could the child have any picture of the female genitals to account for a later horror of them, as Rank assumed. However, Freud was sufficiently impressed with Rank's presentation finally to bring together his own thoughts about anxiety and present them for the first time.[1] Rank saw the sexual act as an effort at symbolic reunion with the mother. (The woman could only achieve this by identification with her unborn child.) Reunion with the mother is the great craving but obstruction to the fulfillment of this is produced by the anxiety of the birth trauma. It is as if in order to return to her this danger must again be encountered. The Oedipus myth, according to his interpretation, is an attempt to solve the mystery of the origin and destiny of man by an attempt to return into the mother's womb. The tragic results of this, depicted in the myth, are seen as expressions of working of the birth anxiety.

As long as these views were merely theoretical and Rank's orientation remained mechanistic and biological, there was lively discussion but no serious cleavage from Freud. However, Rank presently utilized his theory in constructing a new technique of therapy. His aim was to shorten analysis, and he concluded that if every neurosis has its origin in the birth trauma, perhaps analysis can be shortened by utilizing only that problem from the beginning. This he did by setting a definite time for ending the analysis very early in the course of treatment. When he did this, he states, he found that the patients began to have birth dreams. The thought of leaving the analyst, he believed, brought out all the anxieties of birth.

[1] Sigmund Freud, *The Problem of Anxiety*, W. W. Norton & Co., Inc., New York, 1936.

Freud criticized this new departure in technique, saying that it was as if in the midst of a great conflagration one hoped to extinguish the fire by removing the lamp which had caused it.

Rank's new attitude in therapy had one immediate positive result—it brought the analyst and the analytic situation into more prominence than was the case with the Freudian technique. This was the first move towards a better understanding of the analytic situation. Because the analyst was more active, he became a definite force to be reckoned with by the patient, and Rank's interpretation of this fact seems to have led to the next stage of his thinking, in which he discarded the biological orientation altogether and broke completely with Freud's theories. Rank saw the patients all reacting to the threat of separation, and he concluded that people tend to remain dependent, become frightened at the thought of independence and are ready to give up the leadership of their own lives because of the fear. At this point Rank concluded that the patient's problem is really the problem of learning to assert his own will. This was another type of birth, the birth of individuality or will. According to him, people are developed and educated in such a way that they tend to have a sense of guilt whenever they assert themselves. They behave as if they think it is wrong not to submit and conform. The therapist's task is to free the patient from this sense of guilt. He saw the Freudian technique, with its emphasis on the authority of the analyst, as strengthening the patient's tendency to submit, i.e., weakening the patient's will.

Rank instituted three modifications of technique. The first was, like Jung's and Adler's, placing the chief emphasis on the present situation in the analysis in contrast to Freud's emphasis on the past, while treating reactions to the analytic situation as resistance. For Rank the therapeutic process involves a "new experiencing," not merely a re-living of the infantile past. Secondly, with Rank's emphasis on the birth trauma he saw the reaction to the analyst as primarily that to the mother and not to the father. The mother transference Rank actively presented to the patient from the beginning. The third modification was setting a definite time limit to treatment and considering the patient's reaction to that the most important material to be discussed. Of the three modifications the first, making the analysis a living experience in the present with the analyst, is the most valuable. As Jung and Adler had already noted, it presents a new way of looking at therapy, a way to be utilized differently by Ferenczi, Reich and later workers. The stressing of the mother transference had already been brought out by Jung. However, Rank rediscovered it in a new connection. The setting of a termination to analysis proved to be the least satisfactory of his innovations, although it has been found to be a useful idea if used with discretion and flexibility. But in its original rigid form even Rank himself eventually discarded it.

So around 1925 Rank was advocating a more active form of therapy designed to encourage the patient to assert himself and find his own individuality. This was in line with Jung's emphasis on the importance of releasing the patient's repressed potentialities. Rank saw it in terms of will, and with the will and its mode of operation as a measure, he divided people into three types, the "normal" or adjusted, the neurotic, and the creative artist. The "normal" man accepts the popular will as his own. This is seen not necessarily as passive submission; it may be, and when healthy is, an active aligning himself with the will of the group. The neurotic is the one with difficulties—he cannot positively identify himself with the group nor can he stand alone, for standing alone produces a feeling of inferiority and guilt. The creative artist has succeeded in fully accepting and affirming himself. He is in harmony with his powers and ideals. "In a word, with this type . . . is formed neither a compromise, nor merely a summation, but a newly created whole, the strong personality with its autonomous will, which represents the highest creation of the integration of will and spirit." [1] The normal person does not seek treatment—he is adjusted. The creative artist does not need treatment for he has succeeded in affirming himself. The goal of therapy is to bring the neurotic to a point where he can affirm himself and assert his will. It is clear that in Rank's thinking becoming a creative artist is more desirable than becoming "normal."

Rank's idea of will, which plays a central role in his later theories, is often rather vaguely drawn. He saw it as developing primarily as a negative force against compulsion. The compulsion may be from external forces such as parents or the internal demands of sexuality. The danger from sexuality was seen to be that it might impel one to submit to another will. Next, a second more positive level of willing is reached directed towards desiring what others have or want. By this he did not mean envy but a desire for similar aims and ambitions. This is merging one's will with the will of

---

[1] Otto Rank, *Will Therapy and Truth and Reality*, Alfred A. Knopf, New York, 1947, p. 265.

the group. Finally comparisons are given up and positive willing is achieved when a person no longer measures himself by others' standards, but can take responsibility for his own willing. He points out that by education we are given a sense of evil connected with asserting our own wills. This idea comes from training in the necessity to conform in some things.

Rank asserted that the creative artist could not be understood from Freudian theory. Freud leaves no room for positive creativeness but assumes that all that is good in man is the result of the reaction of society in bringing about the sublimation of biological instincts.

In the books following the publication of *Will Therapy* Rank's thinking becomes more confused. There is often an indefiniteness of meaning, making a variety of interpretations possible. This is especially true of his ideas about truth. At one point he states that truth is subjective. "Truth is what I believe or affirm, doubt is denial or rejection." [1] On the same page he states that what is can only be discovered if one overcomes the tendency to deny what one does not want to see. Then he continues, "The third level of creative consciousness or phantasy is the most positive expression of the counter-will, which not only says 'I will not perceive what is but I will that it is otherwise, i.e. just as I want it. And this, only this, is truth.' " [2] Clearly he is talking of different kinds of "truth" and he seems to believe that truth, in the usually accepted sense of what is really so, is something which cannot be endured. So he would seem to conclude that the creative

[1] *Will Therapy and Truth and Reality*, p. 247.
[2] *Will Therapy and Truth and Reality*, p. 247.

artist makes his own truth. When this thinking is applied in therapy, one finds confusing results depending upon the different possible interpretations. Thus the idea of accepting and affirming oneself can be and has been interpreted in two ways. It can mean seeing yourself as you really are, becoming aware of assets and liabilities, with the result that you are freer to develop—the truth has made you free from the false images of yourself. Or accepting oneself can mean saying "I am all right just as I am. I assert my right to be this." Both meanings can be justified from Rank's hypothesis.

The second interpretation tends to glorify rebellion or being different as an end in itself. This is encouraged not only by the confused concept of truth, but also by the stress placed on encouraging the assertion of the counter-will. It also minimizes the necessity of dealing with reality factors in the environment, e.g., other people's wills, etc.

In all active therapeutic procedures the danger of the therapist's appearing to be sadistic is greater than in the more passive methods. Rank's method seems especially to lend itself to this possibility. In encouraging the patient to assert his will, therapists have felt justified in doing or saying things chiefly for the sake of making the patient angry. It was thought that by encouraging rage in the patient, one was developing his independence and will. While Rank's method especially encourages such treatment, he was not entirely alone in thinking there was value in this. In the late 1920's one of the reactions to Freud's discovery that repressed aggression was also an important factor in neurosis was a tendency to feel something important had been accomplished whenever the patient "got out" some rage. More details of this will be discussed presently when considering Ferenczi's contribution.

Another unfortunate aspect of Rank's method of therapy is that it gives no security to the very dependent patient. Psychotics and all people genuinely unable to stand alone can be forced prematurely by his method to attempt to stand on their own feet and make their own decisions. The result often is panic.

So the dangers of Rank's therapy are of two kinds. Too great permissiveness may lead the patient to settle for a compromise or an illusion if he interprets truth in terms of what he wants it to be. The second danger is that the method may be used sadistically and force the patient to take a stand he cannot maintain.

Although the practical application of Rank's thinking seems to have had serious hazards, there are some points of value. Like Jung he asserted that the neurotic had difficulties partly because of inability to express positive aspects of himself. He saw the highest development to be the creative artist, who had become able to express his uniqueness, sometimes without the approval of society. In seeing the neurotic's problem as inability either to conform or express his creative side, he stressed the possibility of developing the potentialities of the patient. His method focused attention on the dynamic possibilities of the doctor-patient relationship. To him cure had to do with the final assertion of the patient's counter-will. When the patient is able to overthrow the authority of the analyst, he is free. This questioning of the power of the analyst he considered an essential part of the growing independence of the patient. He also proclaimed the analyst to be an important figure in his own right in the analysis, not merely a "mirror," and he saw that the analytic situation was something more than a simple repetition of the past. The shift of emphasis from recall of the past to the study of the dynamics of the analytic situation was one of the most important steps in the development of psychoanalysis and Rank contributed to this. He was the first person in the 1920's to attack Freud's "therapeutic nihilism."

FERENCZI

For many years Ferenczi was closely associated with Rank. Both had in common a desire to find an effective therapeutic method, and they collaborated until Rank made his decisive split with Freud. From that point on they developed differently. Both sought for improved therapeutic effectiveness in a better understanding of the analytic situation. However, Ferenczi's approach to the problem was quite different from Rank's. Ferenczi developed his thinking in two phases—first a phase of active technique and later a phase of permissive technique, which he called "relaxation" therapy.

In the active therapy the aim was, like Rank's, to rouse reactions in the patient. Ferenczi, sticking closely to Freud's thinking, based his activity on Freud's dictum that analysis should be carried on in a state of privation. Freud's theory was that the more libido was deprived of outlets of discharge, the greater the amount which could be abreacted in the analysis. Thus he recommended that analysis should be carried on in a state of sexual abstinence. So Ferenczi first worked with the idea that the more the patient was deprived of body pleasures the more emotion would appear in the analytic hour, which, he hoped, would increase therapeutic effectiveness. The patient was therefore urged to give up all sexual satisfaction, to limit the frequency of urination and spend as little time as possible in other toilet activities. Also eating or drinking for pleasure was to be denied. This mode of analysis certainly produced much violent emotion, and for a time he thought it was effective. Eventually he became convinced, however, that the emotion he was observing had little if anything to do with the repressed emotion he was seeking to liberate. The reactions were anger and irritability, which to a great extent were justified by the uncomfortable life situation created by his prohibitions. I have just pointed out in discussing Rank that in trying to make the analytic situation a more genuine emotional experience many analysts in the 1920's felt that the active stirring up of emotion in patients was justified. They were under the mistaken impression that they were thus releasing repressed emotion. If the patient was able to rant and rave against the analyst, he was supposedly freeing himself from his father or some equally important early figure. Abreaction was still considered the method of cure. Ferenczi's experiment showed that deliberate attempts to stir up anger did not produce the desired result. He relinquished his method gradually, that is, he first modified it to the extent of making the undertaking of privation voluntary. He concluded that only if the patient was genuinely willing to undergo this kind of self-deprivation and there was no realistic resentment towards the analyst, were the emotions thus stirred up of therapeutic significance. However, this too did not work well. Many patients out of fear of the analyst's disapproval agreed to the abstinence rule, which they nevertheless resented. So he abandoned the whole method.

Around 1927 he swung to the opposite extreme and developed his relaxation therapy, in which he acted on the assumption that since neurotics were people who had never been accepted or loved as children, their need was to discover the experience of love and acceptance. By furnishing a favorable environment in analysis, he thought perhaps these people could grow up again with a "good parent." How he made this revolutionary about-face is not clear. It is most likely that it grew out of his actual work with patients. He concluded that one reason for the therapeutic success of analysis had been the fact that it furnished the patient with a different environment, an atmosphere of tolerance instead of disapproval, and that because of the *difference* in the new experience from that of the past the patient was able to become aware of the tensions under which he had been living. At this point Ferenczi was in effect claiming that the actual relationship to the analyst is important. Not only can the patient try to relive his past relationships with the analyst, as Freud believed, but because the analyst has a different attitude, the patient also has a *new* experience with him. Jung and Rank had made similar observations although each one of these had emphasized different aspects of the new experience. With Ferenczi, the emphasis was on the attitude of the analyst. Like Jung he believed that children sense and react to the personality of the parents even before they learn the meaning of words. In the very intimate relationship of analyst and patient he assumed some similar mode of awareness must also exist. Therefore every patient reacts to the real personality of the analyst as well as undergoing the experience of transference. He saw the analyst's personality as the instrument of cure. Since no one exists without some defects, he felt that the analyst should openly admit his faults and mistakes whenever they appeared in the analytic procedure. When the analyst denied them overtly or tacitly, they increased the patient's difficulties in two ways. He became confused as to which of his experiences were based on the distortions of transference and which were adequate to and based on the actual situation between him and the therapist. Also, the analyst, by denying having any shortcomings, was actually repeating the authoritative attitude of parents who operated on the premise that they were always right. When the analyst behaves too much like the real parents, Ferenczi thougnt, the patient falls into a reliving of his childhood situation without insight. In short Ferenczi stressed the belief that it was the fact that the analytic experience was different from the patient's past life experience that made it therapeutically effective. The revolutionary kernel in this was the idea that the analyst might, without losing his authority, admit the fact when he had made a mistake or shown some emotional involvement in the situation. Another aspect of Ferenczi's theory about the significance of the real relationship was his belief that the analyst must really like and accept the patient for what he is—shortcomings and all—or no therapeutic situation is possible. It is clear that in this stressing of the importance ot the real attitudes of the analyst, Ferenczi had turned his interests to the study of the interaction of people with one another.

Another innovation of his at this period was that of en-

couraging the patient to dramatize. This seems to have developed from the idea that the patient was to re-live his
childhood with, as it were, a better parent. So he encouraged
the patient to act as if, for instance, he were three years old,
even to the point of talking "baby talk" or playing with
dolls, etc. In this the analyst would participate by treating
the patient like a three-year-old.[1]

In making the analytic situation a living vital experience
Ferenczi still had his eye on the past. It was the past which
was relived in the present—but with a difference. There is
a new element added, namely, the contribution from the
analyst's own personality. There is here also an important
difference between Ferenczi's idea of re-living the past in the
present and Rank's seeing the past as only vital when it becomes the living present. Ferenczi seems to stress the past, as
if it were valuable without regard for its present realistic influence, while Rank's view emphasizes the importance of the
present situation.

Ferenczi's method was criticized severely by Freud, who
especially viewed with suspicion the idea of giving "love" to
the patient. Admitting one's mistakes to patients also seemed
to Freud unwise.

It is my opinion that Ferenczi did not have a clear idea of
neurotic love demands. His assumption that patients fell ill
because they were not loved and accepted as children was a
useful concept, but he thought the adult neurotic's craving

[1] A similar technique has been attempted by John Rosen recently. See
John N. Rosen, "Treatment of Schizophrenic Psychosis by Direct Analytic
Therapy," *Psychiatric Quarterly*, Vol. 21, January, 1947, pp. 3-37; also
"Method of Resolving Acute Catatonic Excitement," *Psychiatric Quarterly*,
Vol. 20, April, 1946, pp. 183-198. Compare also Moreno's psychodrama.

for love was simply a repetition of the unsatisfied childhood longing. He did not see that the neurotic need of love is already serving other purposes such as being a device for concealing hostility or gaining power, etc., and that the longing for love also continues not because none is available but because the patient has become incapable of accepting it. In other words, his early experience has so moulded his character that he cannot utilize love when it is offered. Because of this his demands are insatiable. No matter how much genuine warmth the analyst is capable of giving, the childhood lack in the patient cannot be repaired except through insight-provoking analysis of his character defenses which thwart and block him at every turn. Although Ferenczi did not see this, he soon found that he could not give a patient all the love the latter demanded. Nevertheless, the idea that the analyst must like and accept the patient in order to help him is in a general sense a valid observation.

The idea of admitting mistakes to the patient also must be applied with insight into the patient's needs. It should not degenerate into a mutual analysis because this makes heavy emotional demands on the patient, and with some types of patients, also, the analysis could easily become chiefly an analysis of the analyst. So a middle ground must be found between authoritarian self-righteousness on the one hand and, on the other, placing oneself completely under the control of the patient. This is a difficult position to maintain and Ferenczi did not quite see all the pitfalls. However here, too, is the kernel of a good idea, which Sullivan and Fromm-Reichmann have re-discovered in working with psychotics. It is apparent that some recognition of the limitations of the analyst, the participant observer, is a part of the interpersonal process.

Making the analysis a dramatic reliving of the past has less to recommend it. According to the experience of the writer, with the average neurotic his sense of reality keeps him from genuinely participating. It becomes a kind of mechanical act without sincere emotion. Occasionally in analysis a fragment of the past is re-lived spontaneously with genuine emotion. Only then can it be utilized therapeutically. Moreover, with patients whose sense of reality is already easily disturbed, as in the case of borderline psychotics, encouragement in "acting out" can push the patient further into unreality. Nevertheless Rosen and Moreno report success in utilizing a similar method.

Ferenczi never broke openly with Freud's thinking, but at the time of his death in 1933 his relations with Freud were strained and the latter viewed with consternation much of Ferenczi's "relaxation" therapy.

REICH

In the 1920's Wilhelm Reich also made a significant contribution to a better understanding of the analytic situation. His lectures on technique to the students of the Vienna Institute presented a new type of therapeutic activity. He advocated a frontal attack on the character resistances. This technique, as I have already said, gave the first effective approach to the analysis of character structure. Horney, Sullivan and others have since made improvements on Reich's ideas, but he was the first one to organize psychoanalytic thinking about the subject and even today his lectures, published in *Charac-*

ter Analysis, are still among the best practical guides on the subject for the student. Reich did not question the libido theory. In fact, according to the later development of his own school, one might say he out-Freuds Freud as far as stressing libido is concerned. He did, however, take issue with the concept of the death instinct, as will be discussed presently. Reich's later ideas wander far from the field of psychoanalytic thinking and have not been confirmed by others.[1] I must even question his earlier idea that orgastic potency is a criterion of cure, if he means by this merely physiological performance. It has often been observed that many schizophrenics are capable of this. It would seem that orgastic potency is important as evidence of mental health only when it is integrated with the total personality and expresses full emotional relatedness to the other person.

Criticism of his later thinking, however, should not detract from an appreciation of his earlier contribution, especially in the field of character analysis. Ferenczi had earlier pointed out that tensions and postural attitudes of patients sometimes were expressive of resistance, and that calling the patient's attention to them often resulted in producing significant progress.[2] Reich went into the matter much more extensively. He found body tensions a very frequent mode of expressing emotional states, but in addition he found that people had characteristic ways of reacting which were expressed psychologically as well as in somatic tensions. Some

[1] Some of his experiments have been repeated with negative results by T. Hauschka, senior member, in charge of the Department of Experimental Zoology, The Institute for Cancer Research. (Report shortly to be published.)

[2] Sandor Ferenczi, *Further Contributions to the Theory and Technique of Psychoanalysis,* The Hogarth Press, Ltd., London, 1926, Ch. 15.

people, for example, habitually meet life situations in a passive way. Some have techniques of ingratiating themselves.
Some are aggressive, etc. These he saw as compact protective
mechanisms developed out of the patient's whole past.

What Reich did not grant and what is accepted generally
today is that dealing with these attitudes is part of analysis.
He termed analyzing the character resistances "education for
analysis." He believed that after these attitudes are broken
down by repeatedly calling the patient's attention to them in
all situations, then the analysis itself begins, and here he
thought of analysis, in the traditional manner, as a study of
the vicissitudes of the libido. Probably because Reich still
thought of character traits essentially as resistance, his approach to them was ·more direct and was made probably
earlier in the treatment than is done by most analysts today,
with the possible exception of Horney. Today character
trends are treated like other neurotic symptoms. Insight into
them is to be presented to the patient only when he is ready
for it and can therefore utilize the knowledge constructively.
It is probably because of Reich's more active attack on the
defenses that he warned the student against using the method
with patients who have a great deal of anxiety. This method,
with its active attack on the defense system, is itself anxiety-
producing.

Reich's interest in character led him in the early 1930's to
some important observations on the relation of character and
society. In 1933 he wrote, "In connection with the sociological function of character formation we must study the fact
that certain social orders go with certain average human
structures, or, to put it differently, that every social order

creates those character forms which it needs for its preservation. In class society, the ruling class secures its position with the aid of education and the institution of the family, by making its ideologies the ruling ideologies of all members of the society. But it is not merely a matter of imposing ideologies, attitudes and concepts on the members of society. Rather, it is a matter of a deep-reaching process in each new generation, of the formation of a psychic structure which corresponds to the existing social order, in all strata of the population." [1] His paper on the masochistic character,[2] published in 1932, was the immediate cause of his break with Freud. In this paper he questioned the existence of a death instinct and denied that masochism was an expression of it. He saw masochism rather as (in the final analysis) an adjustment to disastrous social conditions. One must take issue with much of Reich's thinking in this paper and others which he wrote around this period, but his seeing the character structure as created by the social order is one of the early indications of the developing interest in cultural factors in neurotic difficulty.

It is clear from these brief accounts of the work of Rank, Ferenczi and Reich that significant development took place in psychoanalytic technique in the 1920's, and that this brought into new prominence the importance of the analytic situation as a vital experience in its own right, the beginning of interest in the interpersonal process and a relative diminishing of emphasis on the study of the distribution of the libido. Each of the three men in his own way made a

[1] *Character Analysis*, p. xviii.
[2] *Character Analysis*, Ch. xi.

contribution to this development. Also in the 1920's, for the first time American psychiatry came importantly into the picture. Psychiatry in America, under William A. White and Adolf Meyer, had for years been stressing the importance of environmental factors in mental illness. Therefore the men who went from America around 1920 to study psychoanalysis in Europe already had a point of view which must have in many instances modified their approach to Freud's orientation.

chapter ten

RECENT DEVELOPMENTS

It HAS BEEN THE AIM OF THIS BOOK TO TRACE
the course of psychoanalytic development, to point out the
paths which have led in the direction of progress and to
criticize as impartially as possible the theories and experiments which have been unfruitful. Current history always
constitutes the most difficult task in objectivity, especially if
one is describing situations or thinking in which one has
been an active participant. In this respect the present writer
recognizes her vulnerability. She recognizes also that current
discoveries need time for testing and verification and that,
therefore, especially in the field of human behavior, a final
evaluation of the thinking of recent years must wait for a
greater perspective.

In the last chapter I described the significant changes in
the 1920's which resulted in a reawakening of interest in
psychoanalysis as a method of therapy. From bringing the
analytic situation into the foreground of interest, new insights developed and new theories were formulated. I have
stressed chiefly the emphasis placed on the current situation,
especially as observed in the analyst-patient relationship. An-

other influence was beginning to be felt in the late 1920's, namely the findings of modern anthropology and sociology. Especially the study of comparative cultures was beginning to attract the attention of a few analysts. Prior to this time anthropology had been a subject of interest to analysts, but in a different way. The points where the history of primitive cultures had seemed to coincide with analytic theory had been stressed. Analysts had dabbled in the symbolism of primitive rites in terms of psychoanalytic theory without attempting to understand the pattern of the culture. Anthropologists had made little use of the findings of psychoanalysis.

About 1930 a few analysts had begun to show a new kind of interest in anthropological studies of culture, and one anthropologist, Edward Sapir, was a pioneer in advocating collaboration of anthropology, sociology and psychoanalysis.

In the preceding decade many American psychiatrists had gone to Europe to study psychoanalysis. Most of them had not stayed more than a year or two and so had not become completely immersed in the psychoanalytic theories prevalent in Europe. In the 1930's the majority of European analysts were forced to leave Europe, England and the United States becoming the new centers of psychoanalytic development. The war, with its limitation of transportation, its paper shortage, etc., for many years made active collaboration between the two new groups difficult (i.e., England and the United States). In this way European analytic thought and American analytic thought began to fuse while for the time being at least the American and English groups have progressed in different directions. In this book I shall attempt to present only the American contribution.

Since the 1930's American psychiatry has become increasingly important. In the last chapter I pointed out that in general American psychiatrists, with their background of training in the importance of environment as contributing to mental illness, had a tendency to interpret Freud's system less literally than the Europeans did. There were also a few Americans who developed independently of any direct personal contact with the European school. Outstanding among these was Harry Stack Sullivan, who began his study of schizophrenia around 1925. His work challenged Freud's idea of transference because he was able to demonstrate that patients hitherto considered by Freud incapable of treatment because they were narcissistic, could respond to psychoanalytic methods. In his work with psychotics Sullivan also, independently, concentrated much of his attention on what was going on between patient and therapist. Sullivan was from the beginning skeptical of the libido theory and Freud's instinctivistic framework.

By the middle of the 1930's several new interests were well under way. A more active technique was being developed designed to cope with the problem of analyzing character structure. Growing awareness of the importance of the interaction of analyst and patient marked the beginning of the study of interpersonal relations. The scope of therapy was being enlarged to include psychotics and, finally, a few analysts were beginning to think of learning more about the relation of man to his society by a collaboration with anthropologists and sociologists in the study of comparative cultures. In the last project one analyst, Erich Fromm, as I have shown, had much to contribute. However, even today it is a relatively small group of analysts who are interested in developing a science of human relations based on a study of cultures. Four names should be mentioned as definitely contributing to this field: Fromm, Horney, Kardiner and Sullivan. Of these Fromm was one of the earliest and most significant contributors. Horney, greatly influenced by him, made further practical applications of his thinking. Sullivan, who for some years had been seeking a means of rapprochement between psychiatry and the social sciences, joined forces with Horney and Fromm soon after their arrival in America, and at last put into concrete form his dream of creating a school where the distinctive contributions of the related disciplines could be combined. Edward Sapir and Ruth Benedict were among the anthropologists interested. By 1936 this small group was collaborating in studying the interaction of man and his culture. Kardiner at the same time was developing in a similar direction but did not ally himself with the others. Although he has made informative contributions to the study of culture, he seems unfortunately to have been loath to discard some of Freud's terminology and more speculative thinking. As a result, his work sometimes gives the impression that he is trying to make the data fit the theory.

The most significant and most revolutionary of the contributions to psychoanalytic theory and practice are those of Horney, Fromm and Sullivan, and I shall limit my discussion to their work. Horney and Fromm had already exchanged ideas in Europe before they came to the United States. By 1934 they and Sullivan had discovered that they had many interests in common and for several years the three were closely associated. Although each eventually developed in his own way, it is not surprising to find that their similarities are greater than their differences. Nevertheless, there are differences, and the differences are greater between Horney and the other two than are the basic differences between Fromm and Sullivan.

H O R N E Y

Of the three Horney was the first to publish in a comprehensive form her ideas which had crystallized after her arrival in America. In *The Neurotic Personality of Our Time,* published in 1937, she first presented an extensive cultural interpretation of neurosis. In her second book, *New Ways in Psychoanalysis,* she definitely took issue with Freud's biological orientation. This, of course, had previously been done by Adler, Jung and Rank, who had each in turn substituted a new system. Horney also was substituting a new system, a kind of re-evaluation of many of Freud's observations in the light of the findings of the social sciences and her own experience with patients.

Another significant aspect of her thinking is her emphasis on the importance in analysis of the present situation of the patient. Not only does she stress the immediate analytic situation, like Rank, Ferenczi and Reich, but she places great emphasis on exploration of the current life situation. In this her approach has much in common with Adler, although her outlook is not as limited as Adler's. In place of Freud's sexual etiology, Adler substituted the will to power as the basic problem in human beings, and there is no very definite recognition of it as primarily a neurotic force. Horney definitely sees the will to power as a neurotic mechanism and only one of several possible neurotic mechanisms. Thus in her first book she accords the neurotic need of love a comparable significance. I believe that the latter idea was presented for the first time by Horney. That the craving for love itself could have neurotic aspects seems to have escaped the notice of previous analysts. I have already pointed out that confusion about this existed in Ferenczi's mind, and it can be assumed that his was not an isolated case. Horney's active approach to these neurotic trends is very similar to Reich's. In her later books little new is added to her first theoretical formulations, and I shall merely attempt to underline her most important contributions.

She presented a new interpretation of the repetition compulsion. Thus she pointed out that the phenomena included under the term by Freud were not simply mere automatic repetitions of early childhood situations and that these phenomena did not seem to occur in a compulsive manner. The father transference, for instance, was not a carbon copy of the patient's attitude towards his father at the age of four. That early attitude was the base from which attitudes towards authority had developed, but the original attitude had been added to and modified in the course of growing up by subsequent experiences with father figures, and the final transference picture was an end result of all these experiences. Not only were the patient's attitudes changed by his experiences with the different characteristics of later figures, but it was also altered by psychological vicious circles developed within himself. Vicious circles as she describes them grow out of the neurotic defenses developed, in the first place, in order to solve or circumvent difficulties. So if one has adjusted to a difficult father by becoming submissive, being submissive presently becomes a problem, and some sort of periodic aggressiveness may be developed to get around this difficulty, and so on. That is, neurotic defenses produced in reaction to difficulties, in turn produce new difficulties which in turn produce new defenses, so that by the time the patient comes for treatment, a complicated defensive system must be unwound, beginning with the patient's present life situation. Reich also made a similar observation when he said that the character defenses must be removed in layers, beginning with the most recent.

Also she revived with a new emphasis Adler's idea of the importance of the patient's neurotic goals. The patient is sick not only because of what happened to him but because, in coping with it, he establishes goals which, among other things, lead him to pursue false values. One of her most interesting examples of this is the idea of the "Idealized Image." This is the defense of having a false or at least faulty picture of oneself and of one's virtues and assets. The more unrealistic this picture is, the more vulnerable is the person to the vicissitudes of life. Horney's new contribution to Adler's idea lies in the way in which she conceives the neurotic goals to contribute to secondary anxiety. Not only is a neurotic goal a potential source of anxiety because it does not have a sound basis, but often there are conflicting neurotic goals. The pursuit of either one jeopardizes the other. So inordinate ambition operating at the same time with the need to be loved can produce insoluble conflict.

As I have already shown in Chapter 6, the way in which

the pursuit of neurotic goals as described by Horney and the way in which the self-system of Sullivan contribute to the production of secondary anxiety are important new contributions to theory.

The fact that she was among the first to develop in detail a description of some of the effects of cultural pressures in producing neurosis is one of Horney's contributions. The modification of the repetition compulsion along with the concept of psychological vicious circles, and the concept of the anxiety-producing quality of conflicting neurotic goals are primary among Horney's new approaches to therapy. She is weakest in her conception of the basic structure of neurosis and in her concept of basic anxiety. This goes with her relative lack of interest in early childhood.

A furore was created in psychoanalytic circles by the publication of Horney's first two books. Any thorough-going criticism of Freud has often been met with the charge of superficiality. Horney was accused of it, of being Adlerian, of having discarded the real essence of psychoanalysis, etc. Because of such a blanket condemnation, the positive contributions outlined above were overlooked.

She has merited some of the criticism because in her enthusiasm for her new approach she has often given the impression that she considers the past life of the patient of no consequence in itself, since she stresses the fact that talking about the past in analysis can be utilized as resistance to facing current problems. Horney's attitude can be understood as a reaction to her earlier training. She was greatly impressed by the statement of a patient who had had many years of analysis and who gave as a reason for wishing further analysis the fact that there were still two years of his childhood which he could not recall. He was not concerned with current difficulties in living. Horney's attitude towards the significance of a patient's past history in treatment is that its recall is not the goal of therapy. She notes that in the process of gaining insight into the present, memories from the past often occur and give added weight to the new understanding of oneself. Thus the insight, according to her, is acquired first and is not produced by the recall of the past. In short, her emphasis is almost entirely on how the current neurotic trends work and produce difficulties, and she shows little interest in how such trends developed in the first place.

Horney is much more concerned with therapy than with theory, and therefore her ideas should be evaluated primarily as contributions to improvement in therapeutic methods. There is no doubt that the positive points emphasized above are useful here. However, the great emphasis on the present, in therapy, to the relative exclusion of the past has its unfortunate aspect too. It really gives a one-sided picture, a kind of structure without a foundation, and often leaves the patient feeling guilty that he has developed so many "bad" trends for no good reason of which he is aware. That is, the feeling that his life is an understandable continuum growing out of his total experience is lacking. The result of this is often the appearance of a dangerous degree of anxiety in him. To attack a defense system before the patient, through study of the past, has developed enough understanding of its origin to free him from guilt about it, must produce one of two results—either panic, or utilization of a kind of verbal insight which enables him to alter his overt behavior without his making a fundamental personality change. That is, he re-forms and tries to cover up his former defense mechanism with a new defense more acceptable to the analyst and those about him.

Reich had pointed out that a frontal attack on the defense system should be avoided when treating anxious people. The living present is, of course, more frightening than the past. To find out, for example, that one has a tendency to be dis-loyal when already one has a low regard for oneself can make one more desperate and despairing. It can increase the feel-ing, "I am really not much good."

Horney seems to think that patients are always looking for someone to blame for their difficulties. Sullivan and Fromm believe that blaming others has its place. The parents are in a sense to blame for what the child becomes, for his difficul-ties grow out of their attitudes towards him. If the patient can first come to see that what he is today is the inevitable outcome of his life experience, his own burden of guilt for his difficulties is lessened and his own self-esteem correspond-ingly increased. With an improved self-esteem he can then face insight into his present neurotic character. Horney, how-ever, emphasizes the patient's responsibility for his difficulties. This was one of the unfortunate aspects of Freud's biological theory. According to Freud the child becomes ill because of the "evilness" of his own instincts. Horney too says, in effect, we become ill because we get so much satisfaction from our "evil" neurotic goals. In short Horney's excessive emphasis on the present and on neurotic goals is fully as one-sided as an over-emphasis on the past and the search for causes. An understanding of both is essential in therapy. The patient can use discussion of the present situation for resistance just as effectively as escape into the past is sometimes used, especially if talking about the present is done to please the analyst.

Another unfortunate result of Horney's approach, not specifically stated by her but implicit in the procedure, is an over-emphasis on the patient's hostile attitude to the analyst. The analyst is the enemy of the patient's defenses. In the presence of the threat of losing his neurotic pseudo-security, the patient becomes more anxious and hostile, and a struggle for power ensues. This is true but is only part of the picture. If the patient tries to win the analyst's approval, Horney also sees this as a power device and a way of covering up his hostility. Again, this is part of the truth, but there is another aspect to be considered. The desire for approval also has a history in the patient's development.

FROMM AND SULLIVAN

The two men who have contributed most to the understanding of neurosis in terms of cultural pressures and the interaction of people are Fromm and Sullivan, men with very different backgrounds; the former a social psychologist trained in the classical Freudian school, the latter a clinical psychiatrist, whose psychiatric outlook was deeply influenced by the teaching of William Alanson White and Adolf Meyer. In many ways the thinking of Fromm and Sullivan is quite different, but they supplement each other and their basic assumptions about human beings are similar. They both differ from Horney in placing less emphasis on the study of the secondary gains in neurosis and in having more concern with the total personality picture. Both, like Jung and Rank, have an attitude of respect for the patient. Fromm especially has much in common with the best in the two earlier men. For example, they all point out that often some of the best potentialities of the individual remain repressed, and that the problem of therapy is to help the patient become himself. Fromm, however, shows much more clearly than Jung and Rank how destructive cultural attitudes participate in thwarting potentialities. The significance of emotional difficulties in the parent in affecting the growing child first stressed by Jung has been *rediscovered* by Fromm and Sullivan and developed further. Each man has a very different vocabulary, partly the result of their different types of training, but also pointing to different nuances of emphasis and interest.

Although Sullivan was primarily interested in psychiatric therapy and therapeutic technique he developed an essentially new theory of psychiatry, in addition to becoming a major theorist in social psychology. His theories grew out of clinical observation and practice. He possessed to a remarkable degree a gift for understanding what goes on between people, and out of this gift have come many practical suggestions in therapeutic technique.

Fromm, on the other hand, is concerned with ethics as well as with psychological and social theory, and he has written more about some of the problems of society than Sullivan has. Fromm sees man's problem as the "specific kind of relatedness of the individual towards the world and to himself." [1] Sullivan sees man's problem as a problem of interpersonal relations. These two formulations show the difference in emphasis on

---

[1] Patrick Mullahy, *Oedipus—Myth and Complex*, Hermitage Press, New York, 1948, p. 241.

the self in its relation to the world. Fromm talks of discovering the "true self." Under this term he includes all the potentialities of the individual which might be developed in the most favorable social milieu. Sullivan in his theory also assumes the existence of large undeveloped areas in the person, and states that, as the result of unfavorable early experiences, people become "inferior caricatures of what they might have been." Because he does not so immediately concern himself with these undeveloped areas, some have erroneously gained the impression that Sullivan considered man as only a product of interpersonal relations with no basic individual core of personality. Such is certainly not the case. Fromm, however, has been more interested in the philosophy of the nature of man than has Sullivan.

FROMM

Early in his career as a psychoanalyst Fromm took issue with Freud's theory of the relation of man to society. I have already presented a comparison of the two views in Chapter 7. Fromm does not consider the satisfaction of instinct as the central problem in human nature. He points out that man at birth has fewer predetermined courses of behavior than any other animal. This means that his ways of adaptation are not by instinct but by learning and cultural training and that "man's nature, his passions, and anxieties are a cultural product; as a matter of fact, man himself is the most important creation and achievement of the continuous human effort, the record of which we call history." [1] Hence, "The most beautiful as well as the most ugly inclinations of man

[1] *Escape from Freedom*, p. 13.

are not a part of a fixed and biologically given human nature but result from the social process which creates man."[1] In fact man gets into neurotic difficulties as a result of the new needs created in him by his culture as well as because of deprivations and frustration of his potentialities forced upon him by it. Man's lust for power and his yearning for submission, for example, are not basic biological needs but attitudes developed out of the raw material of human nature by a specific culture. When predominating trends in the culture are destructive, the individual in it becomes frustrated and also destructive of himself and others. So man's most compelling problems have to do with the needs his society has created in him. These, not sex or aggression as such, create his greatest difficulties.

Many of Fromm's observations in social psychology and ethics can be utilized in therapy. His study of the development of individuality and the kind of difficulties it has produced, as well as his observations of the effects of culture on personality, are probably his most outstanding contributions to psychoanalysis. The gradual evolution of man in Western society has already been presented in Chapter 7. Today man has finally become aware of himself as a separate entity.

With the growing realization of separateness there comes a sense of isolation and a longing to return to the earlier feeling of solidarity with others. But man cannot return to his original state. On the other hand, he has gained "freedom from" but often he has not acquired "freedom to" develop as an individual. So he uses certain irrational methods of relating back to the group: sado-masochism, destructiveness,

[1] *Escape from Freedom*, p. 12.

automaton conformity. These Fromm calls mechanisms of escape. The sado-masochistic mechanism, which he defines somewhat differently from Freud, presents a situation where one person seeks to lean on the other for support. This interdependence does not have the positive quality of mature love, in which the growth and happiness of the partner is important. It is rather a seeking to get something for oneself. The other person represents a power or authority who can be used. He may be used as a "magic helper" who is supposed to solve everything, or he may be someone whose resources can be exploited. The most extreme form of the sado-masochistic orientation is the one where the inflicting or receiving of physical or mental suffering at the hands of the partner is the specific form of relatedness. Even this kind of living together furnishes some protection from the feeling of isolation and aloneness.

The destructive person tries to cope with his feeling of powerlessness by removing all sources of comparison or competition. Unlike the sado-masochist who needs to keep his victim near him, the destructive person must bring himself to a new isolation involving absolute victory over or annihilation of his enemies. Fromm points out that there can be a rational hate when faced with a threat to life or integrity, but the destructiveness which represents an attempt to solve neurotic difficulties is irrational.

Another mechanism of escape is automaton conformity. Here one adopts blindly the pattern of the culture. One bows submissively to indoctrination and accepts the way to live, to feel, to think, implicitly or explicitly recommended by the group.

None of these mechanisms are productive solutions of the problem of isolation.

In *Man for Himself* Fromm classifies people according to their character patterns, and it becomes clear that there is a certain affinity between the kind of non-productive character and the mechanism of escape chosen. He lists five character types already described in Chapter 3. I think it is apparent that the receptive character, for instance, would be especially likely to look for a "magic helper" and that the marketing character would often tend to automaton conformity. As we have already discussed in the chapter on character, it is important to remember that there are many possible combinations not only of character traits but also that a person may even use more than one mechanism of escape.

Fromm has also made an important contribution to the understanding of authoritarianism. He distinguishes between rational and irrational authority. Rational authority is based on genuine ability and competence. A teacher who is imparting his knowledge to a student is in a position of rational authority but his power will steadily diminish as his pupil acquires the information and/or skills of the teacher. This is the kind of real authority which the analyst has. As his patient develops, his authority diminishes.

Irrational authority is not based on competence but on neurotic need for power. One may have power by being a "magic helper" or from various forms of intimidation. A person turning to irrational authority for security finds strength in identifying with the authoritarian force, be it a person, a group or an idea. Freud's Superego, according to Fromm, represents or is a manifestation of authoritarian power.

Fromm has made a new interpretation of the Oedipus complex based in part on the actual account of the myth but expressing also his experience in therapy. According to the myth Oedipus did not kill his father out of rivalry for his mother. He killed his father (who was unknown to him) because he was obstructing his passage along a certain road. After he had killed his father and solved the riddle of the Sphinx, he became king of Thebes and incidentally married his mother. There is no evidence that he particularly desired her. She simply went with the throne.[1] This version of the myth seems to have provided the groundwork for Fromm's interpretation of the Oedipus complex. He sees the latter as primarily an expression of the child's struggle in a patriarchal society to free himself from the authority of parents who desire to mould his life according to their wishes. In the Oedipus period the child is attempting to emerge from his infantile dependency and become an individual. The sexual aspect may or may not be important, but in any case it is not the cause of the struggle with the father.

Fromm has not written specifically about therapy, and many of his ideas have a much wider applicability than simply as contributions to the theory and technique of psychoanalysis. Nevertheless, they have an important influence on theory and therapy, and it is this aspect of Fromm's thinking which especially concerns us in this book. His careful documentation of cultural influences has brought a new critical judgment to bear on Freud's theory of personality development. I have already mentioned his emphasis on the necessity for

---

[1] For a more complete discussion of Fromm's interpretation of the Oedipus myth see *Scientific American*, Vol. 180, January, 1949, pp. 22-27.

an attitude of respect for the patient, an attitude already indicated in Jung's and Rank's thinking. Fromm points out
that in the course of therapy one often needs to stress the
essential healthiness of some of the patient's tendencies which
had met with the disapproval of his environment. The goal
of therapy is not primarily to make the person adjusted to his
culture but to develop a sense of integrity and a respect for
his true self. All adjustments to the culture which violate a
person's integrity produce guilt and shame and a loss of self-
esteem. Fromm sees a real respect for oneself as essential to
genuine love and respect for others.

The distinction between rational and irrational authority
is another concept entailing revision of some of the former
attitudes in therapy. The analyst must recognize his position
of rational authority in the patient's life, but he must be on
the alert lest his position of power tempt him to have an
irrational authoritarian attitude. The satisfactory termination of treatment should be one in which the analyst is no
longer in a position of authority. The whole course of treatment should be one freeing the patient of any tendency to
"cure" himself by attaching himself to an irrational authority. Fromm also feels that some value judgments are essential
on the part of the analyst. Freud has emphasized that the
analyst must be free from a tendency to condemn the patient,
that he must not have any emotional stake in the kind of person the patient becomes. Fromm would agree with this but
points out that the analyst's convictions about what is good
for man must play some part in his goal of therapy. He
would use value judgments in choosing patients for treatment in the first place. A marked insincerity of attitude in a

prospective patient, for instance, would point to the likeli-
hood of unsuccessful therapy. There are certain dangers in
this approach of Fromm's. A note of moral condemnation
can easily slip in, and one may find oneself sitting in judgment on the patient, although I am sure that Fromm's own
attitude is far from this. This is a subtle and complex
problem, involving not only the patient's difficulties but also
the analyst's system of values. It is, therefore, not easy to
establish a rational criterion in this field. Fromm himself feels
he has not yet adequately clarified this concept.

SULLIVAN

Sullivan is the most empirical of all the psychoanalytic
theorists. As a rule he sticks closely to what can be observed.
In fact, he terms all less empirically verifiable theories doctrines. He is the first person since Freud to offer a systematic
theory of personality development, although in his earlier
work Jung also formulated a somewhat fragmentary theory.
Sullivan calls his the theory of interpersonal relations. He
holds that, given a biological substrate, the human is the
product of interaction with other human beings, that it is out
of the personal and social forces acting upon one from the
day of birth that the personality emerges. The human being
is concerned with two inclusive goals, the pursuit of satisfaction and the pursuit of security. The pursuit of satisfaction
chiefly deals with biological needs, but the pursuit of security
is primarily concerned with and a result of the cultural processes. The two are intertwined. If the cultural milieu interferes to a serious degree in the search for satisfaction, as is
the case concerning sexual activity, for example, in some

groups in our culture, this can, of course, become a problem, but most psychological problems arise from difficulties encountered in the formation of security operations. Security, according to Sullivan, has to do with a feeling of belonging, of being accepted. From birth on certain attitudes of the culture are conveyed to the child through the attitudes of the parents and other significant people who themselves are reacting to the culture. Before the infant understands speech or is aware of himself as something separate from his surroundings, some of the attitudes of those who care for him, especially the mother figure, are conveyed to him through "empathy." Anxiety, anger or disapproval on the mother's part, for example, give the infant a feeling of uneasiness, a loss of "euphoria."[1] Later the child is actively indoctrinated in the ways of his culture and the giving or withholding of approval by the parents is a part of the method of teaching. In other words, approval by the parents and others brings a sense of well-being; disapproval, on the other hand, involves a sense of insecurity, anxiety. Presently the child comes to realize that some of the devices used early for obtaining satisfaction, such as crying when hungry, are not only no longer effective, but actually productive of disapproval. So the pattern of behavior already established must be inhibited with resulting heightened tension of the muscles formerly concerned in the activity. For example inhibition of crying produces tension of the throat muscles. These muscle tensions are an essential condition of the experience of anxiety, which is always related to the interaction with others, to interpersonal relations.

[1] Sullivan uses *loss of euphoria* to describe the earliest feelings akin to anxiety in the infant. See Chapter 6.

Anxiety according to Sullivan is a potent force in the formation of the self, but it is restrictive. It interferes with observation, it diminishes the ability to discriminate and blocks the acquisition of knowledge and understanding. It makes accurate recall of the precipitating circumstances difficult and diminishes the possibility of foresight. In short "when there is anxiety, it tends to exclude the situation that provoked it from awareness." [1] In the attempt to avoid the feeling of discomfort produced by disapproval, the child tends to develop and emphasize those aspects of himself which are pleasing or acceptable to the significant adults. He will focus alertness on those of his performances which bring approval and disapproval. And out of this focusing of alertness the self is evolved. Aspects that meet with disapproval sometimes tend to be "disassociated" and are not recognized by the person as a part of himself. However, not all negative evaluations are disassociated. Some may remain conscious but with the label "this is bad." Thus a person may do a certain thing disapproved of in childhood, be conscious of doing it with the definite feeling "I am bad." Some of his activity is of no special interest to the significant people, and the child himself may or may not be aware of it. Here he may use *"selective inattention."* If the behavior, thus classified, becomes important later to others so that they call his attention to it, he may without great difficulty incorporate it into his self-system.

The *disassociated*, however, cannot be easily incorporated. The existence of this he will continue to deny unless through therapeutic procedure he is able emotionally to experience it

[1] Harry Stack Sullivan, *Conceptions of Modern Psychiatry,* The William Alanson White Psychiatric Foundation, Washington, D. C., 1947, p. 21.

as a part of himself. However, the line between selective inattention and disassociation is not clear-cut, the difference being one of degree only.

It is not the function of this book to present a comprehensive statement of Sullivan's theories. This will require further study of his unpublished writings. A preliminary discussion can be found elsewhere.[1] The development of the theory of the self dynamism with Sullivan's conception of its relation to anxiety, his concept of parataxic distortion and his theory of personality development seem to the writer his most significant contributions to theory.

As indicated above, the self is eventually formed out of the mass of potentialities in the effort to meet with approval and avoid disapproval. The avoidance of anxiety which is at first evoked by disapproval is the most potent force in its formation. Since anxiety is directly the result of the loss of the sense of well-being as determined by the significant people, it is apparent that the trends of the culture determine to a great extent whether the self includes many of the positive potentialities of a person or he becomes an "inferior caricature of what he might have been."[2] In short, the self is made up of "reflected appraisals." "The child lacks the equipment and experience necessary for a careful and unclouded evaluation of himself. . . . Hence the child experiences himself and appraises himself in terms of what the parents and others close to him manifest."[3] If the parents respect and love him, he becomes self-respecting. If their attitude is

[1] Mullahy, *Oedipus—Myth and Complex,* Ch. 10.
[2] *Conceptions of Modern Psychiatry,* p. 27.
[3] Mullahy, *Oedipus—Myth and Complex,* p. 297.

derogatory, the child cannot develop respect for himself. So the self in Sullivan's theory contains both desirable and undesirable features, the proportion of each being dependent especially on the type of early influences contributing to its formation. Moreover, it is a fairly stable organization and includes more than what is conscious at any given time.

This should not be confused with Fromm's concept of the true self as a core of potentialities which may or may not have been developed. The potentialities of the true self, according to his theory, exist from the beginning, whereas in Sullivan's theory the self-system is a product of the desire for approval and the effort to avoid disapproval in experience with others.[1] Sullivan's self-system is a part of the personality which can be observed. One must conclude that Sullivan thinks that transcending the culture is, at the very least, difficult. Man is moulded by his culture, and all attempts to break with it produce anxiety. What can be accomplished are modifications within the general framework brought about by the impact of different personalities. Thus unfavorable attitudes on the part of parents can be somewhat counteracted by the influence of teachers and different experiences with comrades. Eventually in the case of patients the influence of the therapist, as a participant observer, can produce modifications of the self-system.

Interpersonal relations as understood by Sullivan refer to more than what actually goes on between two or more fac-

[1] This does not mean that in Fromm's theory the true self can be realized outside of a cultural milieu. For Fromm the true self embodies all the potentialities whether realized or not. Sullivan while recognizing the existence of undeveloped potentialities includes in his self-system only those which have been at least partly realized or put into operation by cultural experience.

tual people. There may be "fantastic personifications" such as for instance the idealization of a love object, or one may relate to a non-existent product of the imagination, e.g., "the perfect mate." Also one may endow people falsely with characteristics taken from significant people in one's past. An interpersonal relationship can be said to exist between a person and any one of these more or less phantastic people, as well as between a person or group evaluated without distortion.

This brings us to Sullivan's concept of parataxic distortion, which is not identical with Freud's transference, although it includes the latter. Parataxic distortion occurs whenever in an interpersonal situation at least one participant is reacting to a personification existing only or chiefly in his phantasy. This would, of course, include transference of early childhood attitudes towards parents to the current situation. Sullivan suggests that this may happen not only in the therapeutic situation but in all interpersonal situations. In fact one of the important purposes of therapy is to make the patient aware of what is going on between him and others based on distorted identifications. The therapeutic situation is seen as only one example of the general behavior. Parataxic distortion, therefore, would be any attitude towards another person based on phantasy or identification of him with other figures. One of the ways of learning what is true and what is parataxic in thinking or feelings about another is by comparing one's evaluations with those of others. This Sullivan calls "consensual validation." One can thus correct many erroneous ideas; and approach a nearer approximation of the truth. When a person for whose judgment one has respect sees a situation in a different light from one's own approach, one is likely to think further about the matter; there may result a modification of the thinking of both or the one or the other will be seen to be nearer the facts as they are. Of course, occasionally both may be far from the truth. This may eventually be corrected by further validation with others.

Sullivan has presented a theory of personality development which is described in terms of the process of acculturation. He divides growth from infancy to maturity into six epochs. The period of infancy lasts from birth to the maturation of the capacity for language. In this period the empathic relationship with the mother is a most important influence. During this time the infant gradually gets some awareness of the limits of his capacities, and he begins to see himself as a separate entity in the universe.

The second epoch, childhood, extends from the end of infancy to the period when cooperating with compeers becomes a possibility. During the period of childhood extensive indoctrination with the culture's requirements occurs. The clash between some of the child's interests and the wishes of the parents becomes marked. Thought begins to appear.

The juvenile era covers the period of growing cooperation with other children, of learning to yield some of his interests in favor of group solidarity. He also learns to compare himself with others through competition. It is also the beginning of discovering a community larger than the home, a community which sometimes has standards differing from those of the parents on several issues. There is a fear of ostracism and a desire to belong.

The period of pre-adolescence begins some time between the ages of 8½ and 12. Sullivan considers this a most significant period because "there is a movement from what we might call egocentricity toward a fully social state." [1] Here for the first time there is a beginning of the capacity for intimacy. A chum is found. Previously the child had held an interest in no one comparable to the interest he had in himself. With the advent of a chum the welfare and happiness of the other becomes as important as his own. Thoughts and activities are shared, and one can for the first time say that a state of love exists. "When somebody else begins to matter as much as I do, then what this other person values must receive some consideration from me. So it is in the pre-adolescent change that the great controlling power of the cultural social forces is finally inescapably written into the human personality." [2]

The next stage, adolescence, Sullivan divides into three parts, "early adolescence from the first evidences of puberty to the completion of voice change; mid-adolescence to the patterning of genital behavior; and late adolescence to the establishment of durable situations of intimacy." [3] Here for the first time the problems of sexuality as such become very important, and Sullivan points out that in our culture the natural fulfillment of the newly developed capacity is inhibited by the discouraging of premarital sexual performances while at the same time early marriage is becoming increasingly difficult.

[1] *Conceptions of Modern Psychiatry*, p. 19.
[2] *Conceptions of Modern Psychiatry*, p. 23.
[3] *Conceptions of Modern Psychiatry*, p. 28. In later lectures he grouped the first two under early adolescence, thus dividing adolescence into only two stages.

There is much in Sullivan's theory of personality development to recommend it. The earlier stages of adolescence seem
more comprehensively described than the later. It is clear
that Sullivan does not consider sex the sole or even chief
determinant of personality stages, although he does not hesi-
tate to accord it a place when he thinks it is pertinent,
namely, in the period of adolescence. He did not consider
his theory of personality or interpersonal relations as worked
out completely to his satisfaction. The fact that it is entirely
an empirical system imposes certain limits on it. Like Freud,
his theory has been developed chiefly from observations of
people in his own culture.

The fact that Sullivan's theory is an empirical system gives
it a definite value in therapy. In fact he is the only psychoanalyst since Reich to formulate a fairly systematic and co-
herent theory of therapeutic technique. His ideas were
evolved in the first place from the observation of patients,
and what he has to say is directly useful in the patient-doctor
relation. The position of the therapist as a participant observer in the therapeutic interpersonal situation has not only
further clarified the fact that the analyst is part of the picture. It has assigned to him a definite role, that of being detached, not authoritarian. In stressing that the important
findings in therapy have to do with interpersonal activity,
Sullivan definitely stresses the cultural aspect of personality
difficulties. He, however, does not emphasize the current
situation out of due proportion. He is impressed with the
importance of giving the patient an understanding of the
development of his difficulties. Two types of patients especially interested Sullivan, the schizophrenic and the obses-

sional, and he made significant modifications of technique in the treatment of these. From his work with schizophrenics he learned the importance of adopting a more flexible approach. A minor example would be that since many such patients would not lie down on the couch, he discovered that therapy could still be conducted successfully with the patient sitting, standing or walking, when these situations were chosen by the patient. The peculiarities of the therapist also were found to be more disturbing to the psychotic than apparently they were to the neurotic and therefore there was need of greater humility, a greater expertness, and a less authoritarian attitude if one was to hold the confidence of the patient at all. These alterations, which were essential in dealing with psychotics, have proved helpful also with other types of cases. Sullivan was early impressed with the facility of the obsessional to talk beside the point. This, he established, was due to the development of substitutive systems of thought designed to lead the patient away from anxiety-fraught areas. When this was the situation, free association led nowhere. The patient skipped endlessly from topic to topic of irrelevant material. Therefore, the task here was seen to be to keep the patient's attention on important data. This requires active intervention on the part of the therapist, and this means the therapist must have in his own mind as early as possible in treatment a picture of the important trends with which the patient is supposedly dealing and he must keep calling these to the patient's attention whenever he engages in verbal flight.

He saw cure as the gradual elucidation to the patient of what is going on between himself and others, especially pointing out the parataxic aspects, in conjunction with his growing insight. Sullivan recognized the value of occasional interpretation of dreams, but he felt this was generally to be avoided in schizophrenia, and in common with good general analytic technique he looked with suspicion on excessive dream production. I shall close the discussion of Sullivan by again reiterating that he was primarily a clinician. He did not have patience with any theory which was not effective or demonstrable in practical work with patients.

In presenting thus the work of Horney, Fromm and Sullivan I do not wish to leave the impression that these three and their followers are the only culturally oriented analysts. There is a general movement, especially among American analysts, toward greater emphasis on culture and environment than formerly. There is more of a tendency among orthodox analysts to stress that Freud himself did not neglect cultural implications. In other words, the trend of the times is towards an interpersonal orientation. As is usual in changing concepts, a few thinkers are somewhat in advance of others, and it is my opinion that these three constitute the advance guard in this respect.

EXPANSION IN RELATED FIELDS

In recent years there is a growing tendency for other professions which deal extensively with personality problems to adapt the insights and some of the techniques of psychoanalysis to their own work. Social workers were among the first groups to incorporate psychoanalytic ideas in their approach to clients. Psychology is beginning to think more in terms of the total personality and to recognize the contribution of psychoanalysis in this realm. The Rorschach and other diagnostic tests are an outgrowth of the newer thinking. Schools are making more effort to understand and help problem children.

The medical profession is becoming aware of the importance of psychogenic factors in disease and of the necessity of treating the patient as a whole. Out of the collaboration of psychoanalyst and medical man is appearing a new development: psychosomatic medicine. This is a research still in its infancy. It has been frequently pointed out that the term "psychosomatic" is unfortunate because it implies a dichotomy between body and psyche, but no better term has yet been discovered.

The more organized psychosomatic studies began in the late 1920's, although the possible relation of emotions to somatic disease had begun to attract attention as early as 1910. Groddeck's vigorous approach to the problem in the 1920's was the beginning of more intensive studies. He attempted analysis of people suffering from heart trouble, nephritis, cancer and other diseases. In some cases he reported at least temporary improvement. Interest in the subject gradually gained momentum, and by 1940 groups of analysts were exploring and studying the possibilities in this field. Two groups, one led by Franz Alexander, and one by H. Flanders Dunbar, were among the first to report their findings. Today the subject is of interest not only to internists and analysts; neurophysiologists also are attempting to learn the relation of emotions to somatic processes.

Theories about psychosomatic conditions are still for the most part mere hypotheses. There is as yet no useful working theory concerning the position of organic disease in the dynamics of personality. Thinking on the subject today is as naïve as was Freud's approach to understanding neurosis in his early case histories. There seems to be a notion current that a thorough analytic training is not as important for those dealing with psychosomatic problems as for those dealing with character and neurosis. There also seems to be a tendency to assume that the psychogenesis of a disease can be established by some kind of brief psychotherapy, that in fact one may even cure a somatic condition by a few months of therapy on a once-a-week basis. There is, for example, a tendency to assume that, because a certain emotional situation occurred just prior to the onset of a disease, *ipso facto* there is a causal connection. Another fallacy in the present approach is the fact that often there is not a sufficient distinction made between hysteria, functional disease, and organic disease with demonstrable organic findings. For example, if some cases of asthma can be cured by psychoanalysis, therefore all cases of asthma, it is sometimes thought, are psychogenic.

In short, there seems to be a tendency to oversimplify matters. I do not consider myself sufficiently adequately informed on the subject to make an authoritative judgment. In my own experience with patients, organic disease, when present, has proved to be among the most difficult of therapeutic access of any of the aspects of a case. I am of the opinion that organic disease, if or when psychogenically determined, must constitute one of the most rigid character defenses. Often the patients are without demonstrable anxiety and, when anxiety is present, it is frequently associated in the patient's mind only with concern about his physical condition. The chronic organic diseases seem especially frequent in rigid personalities. In turn the organic disease may tend to increase the rigidity. It is impossible to say whether one causes the other or whether the two are inseparably bound together and develop simultaneously. Or of course it is possible there is no connection between the two.

There have been two general theoretical psychoanalytic approaches to the understanding of psychosomatic disease. The earlier thinking followed Freud's ideas of libido distribution. Illness supposedly settled in organs which had become erotized for some reason. Thus, for example, oral receptive people were thought to be more prone to gastric ulcer than other types, and anal types specialized in intestinal disorder. Recently there has been more interest in trying to discover how emotions are actually expressed by the body and what changes occur in the biochemistry and neurophysiology of the body under various stresses. This offers a more fruitful scientific approach.

Clearly we have not yet found all the answers to the way human life operates. In the course of sixty years many things have been discovered, but of course it is necessary to continue investigating. Even in the field to which Freud devoted so much energy, the sexual life of man, we must still feel humble. We have learned a great deal about what his culture does to man's sexual drives, but we cannot separate innate sexual drives from cultural attitudes toward sex.

chapter eleven

THERAPY

$\mathbf{P}$SYCHOANALYSIS BEGAN AS A METHOD OF THER-
apy. In the course of the years it has contributed many insights into human personality and from it a body of theory
has developed. Although there have been excursions into art,
literature, education and the social sciences, the need to find
an adequate therapy for the alleviation of emotional disorder
still remains the central goal of psychoanalysis. When Freud
first began his work, he had high hopes that he had found a
method of cure, but gradually it became apparent that the
task was more complicated than it at first had seemed. In
spite of this, Freud continued to work on the problems of
therapy during his lifetime, and in the last twenty-five years,
as we have seen, there has been a new spurt of interest in
finding effective therapeutic techniques.

After Freud's early description of the use of free association as a means of gaining access to repressed memories,
nothing was written specifically about technique for many
years. In 1905, with the publication of "A Fragment of an
Analysis of a Case of Hysteria"[1] he for the first time dis-

[1] *Collected Papers,* Vol. III, case 1, pp. 138-141.

cussed the role of transference in therapy, and between 1910 and 1920 he wrote several papers on therapy. There was, in general, a reluctance to publishing discussions of technique because of a fear that therapeutic methods would be misused by untrained people. Ferenczi published many short notes on technical observations, and Reich finally published one of the most specific guides to the technique of character analysis that has yet appeared. Technique has been taught chiefly by word of mouth through group and individual discussion. This makes the subject difficult for the historian to pull together.

Any discussion of method cannot be divorced from a consideration of the goals of therapy. In over-simplified medical terms, the goal of treatment is cure. But in dealing with mental and emotional problems cure also needs to be defined, and in the last sixty years psychoanalytic thinking has changed about the nature of cure and the goal of therapy. These changes have grown out of discoveries made in the process of treatment.

The first conception of cure was, simply, that it is the alleviation of symptoms, and this was the goal of therapy prior to 1900. The method used during the early years grew out of hypnosis. The patient reclined on a couch and was urged to let his mind wander and to report faithfully everything which occurred to him. Since he was in a doctor's office and had come for treatment of a specific difficulty, his thoughts at first were usually definitely related to his problem. There was a thread of continuity running through his apparently random ruminations, and usually the ideas expressed all had some relevance to his problem. In this way, the patient gradually worked his way back to the recollection of significant episodes which had been fraught with emotion, an emotion or emotions which for one reason or another he had not experienced fully or carried into appropriate action at the time of the event. Very often as the result of this recall, along with the more adequate experiencing of the appropriate emotions, the symptoms of which the patient was complaining disappeared. It seemed to Freud that the method acted like a catharsis, that a quantum of energy which had somehow been "bound" in a symptom was released and that this accounted for the alleviation of the suffering. For many years this "free association" was the only means of access to unconscious material. Dreams were often found helpful as starting points of association. Freud then believed that these all represented expressions of forbidden sexual wishes. This was in line with his conviction that there was a sexual difficulty at the base of every neurotic condition.

Some patients proved to be more difficult to cure than others. Not only were there periods in which nothing important occurred to them, but sometimes recall of apparently meaningful memories did not result in disappearance of the symptom. Concerning the former dilemma, Freud developed his theory of resistance already described in Chapter 5. In many of the latter cases resistance might be a factor; but he also found that at times the failure to improve was due to the fact that more than one memory was involved. He discovered that by continuing to press the patient for further associations, earlier episodes came to mind, that these earlier episodes had similarities or points in common with the later experience, and that the patient's symptom did not disappear until the whole associated network of experiences had been recalled. While the goal of therapy still remained the alleviation of symptoms, Freud now concluded that difficulties early in life were very important contributors to later illness, that, in fact, emotional disturbance in adult life occurred only when a situation arose which corresponded to an early repressed disturbance or its effects. The later situation reactivated the earlier experience, which, then, in attempting to return to consciousness, produced the symptom.

I have already shown how the growing awareness of the importance of early childhood led to significant changes in theory and a shift of emphasis from interest in traumatic experiences to an interest in the course of the biological development of the child. At about the same time the goal of therapy was changed. It was now not enough to note that a symptom had disappeared. One was no longer satisfied unless the "infantile roots" had been uncovered. This meant much more concern with the complete life history of the person. The therapist became a little more active. He called the patient's attention to the importance of early childhood and offered some interpretation of the present in terms of the past. At the same time, almost in contradiction, free association became more "free." The patient was not merely urged to think of his symptom and relate whatever occurred to him; he was given free rein to talk about anything which was uppermost in his mind. Dream interpretation, which for a time had been almost a ritual for beginning the analytic hour, assumed a place of less importance. Freud advised in 1912 [1] that the complete interpretation of a dream in analysis

1 *Collected Papers*, Vol. II, Ch. 27.

was often not only not necessary but definitely contra-indi-
cated, that it might take the patient into areas he was not yet
prepared to meet. He recommended that a dream be treated
like all associations in analysis, that the patient should utilize
his dream material spontaneously in free association and not
be pressed for a complete interpretation. Freud wisely observed that whatever was not dealt with in regard to one
dream would appear again either in some other connection
or in a later dream. It was even discovered that discussion of
dreams could be utilized by the patient as resistance, that is,
as a way of avoiding something more important.

From 1900 to around 1920 the emotional reliving in analysis of past situations was considered to be the way in which
repressions were released. The patient was ill because a part
of his libido had been cut off from free expression by being
"bound" in a repressed memory. When the memory was
made available, the libido was somehow freed and the patient
could now adjust to his current reality. This was cure. There
was some beginning awareness that a neurosis involved more
than symptoms, that there were in the character, for instance,
fixations and regressions which provided, Freud thought, a
part of the constitutional substrate. At that time he thought
very little could be done about this constitutional part therapeutically. It was still believed as late as 1920, and by some
therapists even later, that when the patient had, as it were,
repeated his childhood situation in the analysis with the
analyst, and that when the infantile amnesia had been completely removed, with the appropriate affects accompanying
the recall, the patient should be cured. Unfortunately, frequently no such result was obtained. When the method failed

it was assumed that either the recall of childhood was not complete and that there were still amnesias, or the recall had not been accompanied by adequate affect. The latter situation seemed to be especially frequent in what had come to be called character disorders, i.e., difficulties in living of patients without overt symptoms, who, nevertheless, had general personality problems. Another possible interpretation of failure of therapy, an interpretation which is still accepted by some therapists, was what was called the "negative therapeutic reaction." According to this idea, the patient did not improve in spite of insight because of his masochistic character and his need for punishment. This theory is very complicated and I shall not go into it here except to say that it seems to me to be in some way begging the question since the need for punishment also should be examined analytically. Anyway, around 1920 there was a growing feeling of pessimism about psychoanalysis as a method of therapy. Its effectiveness seemed definitely limited to a few types of conditions.

In Chapter 5 I have discussed resistance and transference. The phenomena observed in patients under these two headings are of vital importance in the dynamics of therapy, and they have received a great deal more consideration since the 1920's. As I have already described, Freud early discovered something of the working of transference and resistance, and he noted that the two were interrelated. He first thought that the patient's tendency to get involved with him was due only to the transferring of childhood feelings and attitudes towards the parents to the analyst, and that all feelings towards him were of this nature. This transference could constitute a very important resistance while at the same time it was also an important source of insight. He saw that it was a resistance in that the patient, by becoming concerned with his relation to the analyst, showing curiosity about him, seeking his love or competing with him, seemed to lose interest in his own problems. In fact, the desire for the analyst's approval, for instance, often inhibited the patient in mentioning some thoughts which, the patient consciously feared, might give the analyst an unfavorable impression of him but which actually would provide more data and perhaps insight.

On the other hand, when it became clear that recall of the past had greater therapeutic value when it was accompanied by appropriate emotion belonging to that past experience, it was then seen that the inevitable concern with the analyst was a part of experiencing the appropriate emotion. The patient tended to *transfer* to the analytic situation the attitudes and feelings concerned with his earlier difficulties, and, through acting them out in the present situation, that is, reliving them, the patient experienced insight into his original problem. Freud thought that too much "acting out" was bad, that one should strive to substitute verbalization for "acting out" whenever possible, but that to some extent some involvement with the analyst was inevitable. Ferenczi greatly clarified this rather confused problem. The problem, briefly expressed, was this. If emotional reliving is essential to cure, why is too much "acting out" to be avoided and at what point is the "acting out" "too much"? Ferenczi concluded that "too much" acting out occurred when there was countertransference. The patient tends to get involved in his own reliving of the past. If the analyst happens to correspond in temperament and attitude to the original significant figure in the patient's life or if the analyst has some "blind spot" (i.e., some personal emotional difficulty of which he is unaware) which is similar to a problem found also in the original significant figure—presumably in most cases the father—the patient gains no insight from the "acting out." He goes on doing what he originally did with a person who, without understanding what he is doing, reacts as the father did. Neither of them, therefore, can become aware of what is going on. Only when the analyst presents a different picture from the original one is the "acting out" profitable. Thus, if one expects all father figures to be stern and authoritarian, and the patient proceeds to react as if this were the fact with the analyst, the absurdity of his cringing subservient attitude or his hostile, defiant one can be seen if the analyst is not stern or authoritarian, but the nature of his behavior remains unnoticed by both patient and analyst when the latter actually has authoritarian tendencies. Ferenczi concluded that the fact that the situation is *different* with the analyst is what makes the patient aware of the original problem and makes it possible for change to take place. Ferenczi, in his thinking, still subscribed to the theory of cure accepted prior to 1920 to this extent, that he considered the emotions appearing in the analysis as simply emotions transferred from the past. It was still a question of releasing old buried feelings, but he had introduced a new point, already indicated by Jung, that the personality of the analyst is important.

Since the middle of the 1920's there have been great changes in therapeutic technique, in the goal of therapy and in the concept of cure. A growing awareness that the analyst's personality plays a part in the picture no matter what he does to conceal it has led to greater insistence that the analyst understand himself as thoroughly as possible through being analyzed. There is a tendency to greater activity by the therapist. Fromm-Reichmann in the middle 1930's expressed the opinion that this activity was possible because by then a great number of cases had been analyzed so that it was no longer necessary to maintain that each new case was a completely new experiment. The analyst, profiting from his knowledge of more or less similar cases in the past, could know that certain types of problems usually had certain types of history and that one could actually help the patients by leading them to the pertinent topics and discouraging endless wandering in unfruitful fields (interminable "free associating"). Reich's approach to character problems represents another form of activity introduced in recent years. His method of pointing out to a person his characteristic ways of relating to others was further developed by Horney and Sullivan and has proved effective with difficult character problems.

Other changes in technique are related to the more active type of therapy. According to the earlier method the analyst generally permitted the patient's transference relationship to him to develop extensively, especially if it were the so-called "positive" transference, before he made any attempt to make the patient aware of what was going on. Freud thought this had to be done in order to bind the patient sufficiently to the analyst so that he would continue in treatment when the situation became less pleasant. When signs of dissatisfaction began to appear, the "honeymoon" was over and the analyst must begin to "interpret" the transference. Today it is clearly seen that this passive nurturing of irrational hopes unnecessarily strengthens the patient's tendency to become dependent on the therapist. Therefore, as soon as any given way of reacting becomes clear to the analyst, first perhaps from studying or observing the patient's activities with his (the patient's) associates and soon by seeing evidences of the same activity in the analytic "me-you" relationship, it can become a topic of discussion. The discussion, of course, must be carried on with tact and a sensitivity for the right moment, but an extreme degree of involvement without insight is seen as not only not necessary but actually harmful in that, among other things, it favors the prolonging of neurotic struggles.

Another change introduced by a few analysts is that of decreasing the number of hours per week required for treatment. Originally it was thought that six times a week was essential in order thoroughly to immerse the patient in the contemplation of his problems. His analysis presumably then became for a period his whole life. When analysis developed in the United States, I suspect that the tendency to take long week-ends contributed to the decision that analysis could be done five times a week. But whatever motive brought the change about, the change itself demonstrated that five times a week still produced effective analysis. The recent war with its great shortage of psychoanalysts, coupled with an increased demand for treatment, has encouraged further experimentation with fewer hours per week, and it has been found that effective psychoanalysis can be done in many cases on a three-times-a-week basis—in very rare cases even on a once-a-week basis. It seems probable that there are different optimums for different patients and this should, of course, be taken into consideration.

The three-times-a-week experiment is responsible for another discovery. In actual duration of treatment, in terms of months and years, the patient going five times a week takes about as long to be cured as the patient going three times. In other words, it is not that the patient only requires a great many hours of talking and discussing of his problems in order to change, but that he seems to require the passage of time in order to consolidate his new insights and incorporate them as a part of his daily living. The repeated testing out and seeing over and over again what is going on seems to be the prerequisite for the process of growth and change. This is what makes treatment so long no matter what method is used. Two practical results of the three-times-a-week method are apparent. More patients can be treated and the monthly cost of therapy is less per person. A prevalent current misunderstanding about the three-times-a-week method should be corrected. Many people seem to be under the impression that regular analytic procedures are not used, that it is not true psychoanalysis but a form of brief psychotherapy. As I have already pointed out, the duration of analysis is not necessarily shortened or lengthened and the method is essentially the same. There is possibly this difference in some cases, that with less frequent contact with the analyst, more of the analysis goes on outside the immediate analytic situation (that is, progress is made through self-analysis, consolidation and incorporations of insight), and there is less unnecessary strengthening of dependency. However, there are patients with limited capacities for self-observation. With these more frequent sessions are indicated. Frequent sessions are also recommended when the patient is in a state of marked anxiety.

As I have already mentioned in discussing Sullivan's contribution, today greater flexibility is permitted in the analytic situation itself. If the patient, for example, makes more rapid progress sitting up, this may well be the best method for him. Insisting that the patient lie down may strengthen his tendency to make the analyst an authoritarian figure. The position itself can be experienced as an expression of submission. Also, lying down enables some patients to keep a feeling of distance and avoid considering their relation to the analyst. With a suspicious, distrustful patient, on the other hand, when he spontaneously lies down, it is usually a sign of confidence and trust in the analyst. It is important only to know why he sits up, why he lies down, why he must watch the analyst or why he cannot look at him. In these details, also, changes often occur in the course of treatment as the result of growing insight. However, it is not the aim of this book to discuss in any detail the technical methods of therapy. I wish only to point out that as the goal of therapy has changed, the method of approaching the patient has also changed. The two are definitely inter-related.

Around 1925 there was evidence that the goal of therapy was changing; in the years since then much thought has been given to the nature of cure. Rank made the observation that the past was important only as it was experienced as a vital part of the present. In other words, a patient becomes ill not because he had terrible experiences in childhood but because these experiences are still active factors in his life. For example, a person is unhappy not because he was unloved in childhood but because this early experience has contributed to making him unable to love and be loved as an adult. A patient can be considered well only when he has become adequately effective in the living present. Thus, a patient who has apparently uncovered all of his childhood repressions and still can not make friends at the present time is not "cured." As has already been pointed out, the new emphasis on the current situation in getting the patient to observe how he is himself contributing to his present difficulties in living has made an accurate observation of the analytic situation important. Instead of one's emphasizing that in the analytic situation the patient relives his past, the analytic experience has come to be seen as an interpersonal situation where the ways in which the patient contributes to his current difficulties in living become manifest and clarified. In this "participant observation" the patient and therapist are concerned not only with the history of the patient's personality difficulties but with their dynamic operation and function in his present way of living. He must become aware of how patterns which produce success and patterns which result in failure have become a part of his way of life. He must learn also the methods by which he distorts what is going on between himself and the important figures in his life. Some of the patient's distorted attitudes in relationships can be explained in terms of Freud's concept of transference, but distortions also occur from projections of the patient's own difficulties. For example, a patient who feels hostile toward most people may assume that other people are equally hostile. Distortions may also occur from the need to carry out a phantasy. If the patient, for example, is seeking a "magic helper," someone who will be a benevolent authoritarian influence in his life, he will endeavor to imagine he has found the essential qualities in the therapist or some other significant person in his present environment. To all of these neurotic ways of relating to people, Sullivan has given the name parataxic distortion. The goal of therapy is the removal of parataxic distortion with the eventual integration of a new type of interpersonal relation more in harmony with the facts as they are. Such a goal does not overlook the importance of the history of trends and difficulties. Each distortion must be thoroughly understood, in respect not only to its goal and the way it operates but also to the way in which it developed. A person is "cured" of a parataxic distortion when it no longer operates in his relationship to people. It is not enough that he consciously stop acting in this or that way; there should be a spontaneous cessation, partly because of understanding, partly because he no longer has any impulse to react in the old way. This means there is no longer any anxiety aroused by failure to conform to the old pattern. This is true insight.

Throughout the years of the development of psychoanalysis obviously there has been a constant effort to define insight. At first it was seen as the result of a mechanical draining off of libido which had been "bound"; next it was thought to be due to an adequate emotional reliving of a past experience. At the present time there has been further clarification. In the three papers on the subject by Eliot Dole Hutchinson[1] one finds a useful working description. He equates insight with the process of creative thought. He sees

[1] *A Study of Interpersonal Relations*, pp. 386-446.

it developing in four essential stages. The first is a period of preparation. Knowledge is acquired, preliminary work is done. There is random trial and error activity calling on ever wider resources and experience. Then comes a stage of renunciation or recession. One despairs of finding the solution; there is a feeling of failure and inferiority; and because the feeling of frustration is unbearable there is usually a shelving of the whole project. The mind temporarily turns to other things. From time to time thoughts about the problem occur and slip away again. Eventually there comes a moment of insight "usually unpredictable in time, though determined by circumstances. This insight consists of more than a simple reorganization of the perceptual field, a new alignment of possible hypotheses. It is often accompanied by a flood of ideas. . . . Noteworthy in this experience are . . . the emotional release, feelings of exultation, adequacy, finality. The period is integrative, restorative," etc.[1] The fourth stage is the period of verification, elaboration or evaluation. This is the period of checking the insight with reality. Sometimes secondary insights develop in this period.

The agent which occasions the insight often seems to be accidental, and there are two types of such experience. The accident may be some experience or event which is related to the problem and is at once incorporated as part of the work. Or the event is not part of the final product and has acted merely as a catalytic agent in the presence of which the other ideas fuse.

These ideas can be applied directly to insight in psychoanalysis. There is the period of working on the problem. The

---

[1] *A Study of Interpersonal Relations*, p. 398.

difficulties are stated and documented. An ever increasing volume of knowledge about them is collected. Speculations are presented by the patient or analyst as to the possible dynamics. For a long time these speculations seem to be merely words. The patient will say, "It sounds reasonable," or "I think that must be the case," but nothing seems to happen. The patient feels just as uncomfortable—he often becomes very discouraged. He may turn his attention to relatively unimportant topics. The problem remains in the background. Then suddenly one day the analyst makes just the right remark or the emotional rapport between the two is especially good—perhaps the patient has just unburdened himself of some doubts or antagonism toward the analyst which the analyst accepts without rancor. This produces a situation with catalytic effect. Then suddenly all the previous thinking falls into place. The patient has the experience of insight. This moment is usually accompanied by a rush of corroborative memories of past and present experience, which result in a general clarification of the subject. Sometimes the insight occurs outside of the analytic situation. An experience may suddenly throw into sharp focus some way the patient is reacting and he sees, experiences, and understands clearly for the first time something which he may have been talking about for months. After this experience the test of the insight's validity should be an effortless change of attitude. For example the patient may report, "Yesterday I was talking to my father and suddenly I realized there was none of the tense, irritable feeling I usually have when I am with him." That is, a change has occurred unconsciously. The calm self-possession is spontaneous; no effort of conscious will is needed. A new interpersonal situation has been integrated.

Why knowing the truth makes you free is open to philosophical speculation. Much more than the animals, the human being seems able to learn from new experience and actually change his ways of adaptation. When a complicated character pattern is clearly brought into awareness and the various defensive attitudes related to it are seen to be no longer necessary for security, that in fact they often contribute to insecurity, man seems to be able to utilize constructively the knowledge for more effective living.

This brings up the important question of what is cure in psychoanalysis. It has been envisioned differently at different times in the last sixty years. Originally cure meant the relief from symptoms. Later, making conscious and experiencing emotionally as much of the repressed as possible was considered essential to furthering permanent relief from neurotic suffering. Today in addition to relief from neurotic suffering a person is considered cured when he is capable of relating to other people with a minimum of parataxic distortions in his behavior and when he is free to develop his powers as far as his education and life circumstances permit. The second arises out of the first. When the life situation is good and the culture predominantly constructive, the healthy person achieves relationship to the group free from neurotic dependency. When the culture is less favorable, he may have to acquire the ability to endure relative isolation. Cure is not synonymous with conformity, nor with happiness as happiness is conventionally understood. A person may remain healthy in adverse circumstances in which he is suffering if he does not have to blind himself to his situation by the various escape mechanisms of neurosis.

It is obvious that absolute cure does not exist. We live in a sick society with which we must make some compromise, and probably no one exists who is so healthy that he can make all the compromises necessary for survival without occasionally resorting to mechanisms of escape, or at least temporary denials of reality. A successful analysis does not offer a person a heaven on earth, as many patients hope. It merely makes it possible for the individual to cope with life with a minimum of psychological excess baggage, that is, repressions, feelings of inferiority, of anxiety, and so on. It is not enough that the patient decide he is cured, nor is it enough that the analyst come to that conclusion, for the human personality is so complicated that no one can be sure that he understands himself or another person completely. The decision to stop treatment should be by mutual agreement with the realization that life may yet stir up more difficulties which can then be coped with as they arise.

It is frequently asked how one can account for the fact that in mental and emotional disorder cures are reported by every psychoanalytic school. Obviously some patients accept their analyst's theoretical formulations as a new form of religion. They "lose" themselves in a new ideology, thus hiding from themselves and others the fact that they have not been cured. This accounts for some, usually the most enthusiastic, recruits. But there are also other types of cures. Many patients achieve deep and lasting insight under or in spite of the various doctrines taught them, if in the interpersonal experience with the analyst the patient's genuine problems in living have been explored. Sullivan has remarked that there is a very strong drive towards mental health in most people. This means they will utilize whatever help is available. Cure is, therefore, not necessarily a sufficient criterion of the truth of the theory used in bringing it about. The history of medicine is filled with evidences of successful treatment in spite of a cumbersome theory. Inaccurate theory is, however, a handicap to the therapist. It circumscribes his thinking and often leads him to pursue unfruitful paths. In this book I have attempted to present the positive and negative aspects of the various theories and methods, keeping clearly in mind that psychoanalysis is still a science in its infancy and no school can lay claim to having discovered the final truth.

BIBLIOGRAPHY

ABRAHAM, KARL

Selected Papers on Psychoanalysis, translated by Douglas Bryan and Alix Strachey, The Hogarth Press, Ltd., London, 1927.

ADLER, ALFRED

The Neurotic Constitution, authorized English translation by Bernard Glueck, M.D., and John E. Lind, M.D., Moffatt, Yard & Co., New York, 1917.

A Study of Organ Inferiority and Its Psychical Compensation, authorized translation by Smith Ely Jelliffe, M.D., Nervous and Mental Disease Monograph Series, No. 24, New York, 1917.

ALEXANDER, FRANZ

Psychoanalysis of the Total Personality, the Application of Freud's Theory of the Ego to the Neuroses, authorized English translation by Bernard Glueck, M.D., and Bertram D. Lewin, M.D., prefatory note by A. A. Brill, Nervous and Mental Disease Publishing Company, New York, 1930.

BENEDICT, RUTH

Patterns of Culture, Houghton, Mifflin Co., New York, 1934.

DUNBAR, FLANDERS

Emotions and Bodily Changes, A Survey of Literature on Psychosomatic Interrelationships 1910–1945, Columbia University Press, 1945.

FERENCZI, SANDOR

Sex in Psychoanalysis, authorized translation by Ernest Jones, M.D., Richard G. Badger, Boston, 1916.

Further Contributions to the Theory and Technique of Psychoanalysis, compiled by John Rickman, M.D., authorized translation from the German by Jane Isabel Suttie, M.A., M.B., Ch.B., and others, The Hogarth Press, Ltd., London, 1926.

FREUD, ANNA

The Ego and the Mechanisms of Defense, translated by Cecil Baines, The Hogarth Press, Ltd., London, 1937.

FREUD, SIGMUND

The Basic Writings of Sigmund Freud, edited by A. A. Brill, The Modern Library, Random House, Inc., New York, 1938.

A General Introduction to Psychoanalysis, authorized English translation with a preface by Ernest Jones and G. Stanley Hall, Garden City Publishing Co., Garden City, N. Y., 1943.

Totem and Taboo, Kegan, Paul, Trench & Trubner, Ltd., London (no date).

Three Contributions to the Theory of Sex, Nervous and Mental Disease Publishing Company, New York, 1930.

New Introductory Lectures on Psychoanalysis, translated by J. H. Sprott, W. W. Norton & Co., Inc., New York, 1933.

Selected Papers on Hysteria and Other Psychoneuroses, authorized translation by A. A. Brill, Nervous and Mental Disease Monograph Series, No. 4, 1920.

Collected Papers, 4 volumes, The Hogarth Press, Ltd., London, 1924.

Beyond the Pleasure Principle, Boni & Liveright, New York (no date).

The Ego and the Id, The Hogarth Press, Ltd., London, 1935.

The Problem of Anxiety, translated from the German by Henry Alden Bunker, M.D., W. W. Norton & Co., Inc., New York, 1936.

Group Psychology and the Analysis of the Ego, authorized translation by James Strachey, Boni and Liveright, New York (no date).

The Future of an Illusion, The International Psycho-Analytical Library, No. 15, 1943.

Civilization and Its Discontents, Jonathan Cape & Harrison Smith, New York, 1930.

"Analysis Terminable and Interminable," *The International Journal of Psycho-Analysis*, Vol. XVIII, October, 1937.

Moses and Monotheism, translated by Katherine Jones, Alfred A. Knopf, New York, 1939.

An Outline of Psychoanalysis, authorized translation by James Strachey, W. W. Norton & Co., Inc., New York, 1949.

FROMM, ERICH

Escape From Freedom, Farrar & Rinehart, Inc., New York, 1941.
Man For Himself, Rinehart & Co., Inc., New York, 1947.
"The Oedipus Complex and the Oedipus Myth," *The Family: Its Function and Destiny,* Vol. V, The Science of Culture Series, edited by Dr. Ruth Nanda Anshen, Harper & Brothers, New York, autumn, 1948.

FROMM-REICHMANN, FRIEDA

"Recent Advances in Psychoanalytic Therapy," *A Study of Interpersonal Relations,* edited by Patrick Mullahy, Hermitage Press, Inc., New York, 1949.
"Remarks on the Philosophy of Mental Disorder," *A Study of Interpersonal Relations,* edited by Patrick Mullahy, Hermitage Press, Inc., New York, 1949.

GREENACRE, PHYLLIS

"The Predisposition to Anxiety," *The Psychoanalytic Quarterly,* Vol. X, 1941.

HORNEY, KAREN

New Ways In Psychoanalysis, W. W. Norton & Co., Inc., New York, 1939.
The Neurotic Personality of Our Time, W. W. Norton & Co., Inc., New York, 1937.
Self Analysis, W. W. Norton & Co., Inc., New York, 1942.
Our Inner Conflicts, W. W. Norton & Co., Inc., New York, 1945.

HUTCHINSON, ELIOT DOLE

"Varieties of Insight in Humans," "The Period of Frustration in Creative Endeavor," and "The Nature of Insight," *A Study of Interpersonal Relations,* edited by Patrick Mullahy, Hermitage Press, Inc., New York, 1949.

JACOBI, JOLAN

The Psychology of Jung, translated by K. W. Bash, with a foreword by C. G. Jung, Yale University Press, New Haven, 1943.

JUNG, CARL G.

"The Association Method," *The American Journal of Psychology*, Vol. XXI, No. 2, April, 1910.

The Theory of Psychoanalysis, Nervous and Mental Disease Monograph Series, No. 19, New York, 1915.

"On Psychological Understanding," *Journal of Abnormal and Social Psychology*, 1915.

The Psychology of the Unconscious, authorized translation with introduction by Beatrice M. Hinkle, Dodd, Mead & Co., New York, 1927.

Two Essays on Analytical Psychology, authorized translation by H. G. and C. F. Baynes, Dodd, Mead & Co., New York, 1928.

Psychological Types or the Psychology of Individuation, translated by H. Godwin Baynes, Harcourt, Brace & Co., New York, 1926.

Modern Man In Search Of A Soul, translated by W. S. Dill and Cary F. Baynes, Harcourt, Brace & Co., New York, 1933.

Psychology and Religion, Yale University Press, New Haven, 1938.

The Integration of the Personality, translated by Stanley M. Dell, Farrar & Rinehart, Inc., New York, 1939.

KARDINER, ABRAM

The Individual and His Society, Columbia University Press, New York, 1939.

The Psychological Frontiers of Society, with the collaboration of Ralph Linton, Cora Du Bois and James West, Columbia University Press, New York, 1945.

MALINOWSKI, BRONISLAW

Sex and Repression in Savage Society, Harcourt, Brace & Co., New York, 1927.

MOLONEY, JAMES CLARK

The Magic Cloak, a Contribution to the Psychology of Authoritarianism, illustrated by Erle Loran, Montrose Press, Wakefield, Mass., 1949.

MULLAHY, PATRICK

Oedipus—Myth and Complex, Hermitage Press, Inc., New York, 1948.

RANK, OTTO
The Myth of the Birth of the Hero, authorized translation by Dr. F. Robbins and Dr. Smith Ely Jelliffe, Nervous and Mental Disease Monograph Series, No. 18.
The Trauma of Birth, Harcourt, Brace & Co., New York, and Routledge and Kegan Paul, Ltd., London, 1929.
Art and Artist, translated by Charles Francis Atkinson, Alfred A. Knopf, New York, 1932.
Will Therapy and Truth and Reality, authorized translation with a preface and introduction by Jessie Taft, Alfred A. Knopf, New York, 1947.

RANK, OTTO, and FERENCZI, SANDOR
The Development of Psychoanalysis, authorized English translation by Caroline Newton, Nervous and Mental Disease Publishing Company, New York, 1925.

REICH, WILHELM
Character Analysis, Principles and Technique for Psychoanalysts in Practice and in Training, translated by Theodore P. Wolff, Orgone Institute Press, New York, 1945.

RIOCH, JANET MACKENZIE
"The Transference Phenomenon in Psychoanalytic Therapy," *A Study of Interpersonal Relations,* edited by Patrick Mullahy, Hermitage Press, Inc., New York, 1949.

ROSEN, JOHN N.
"Treatment of Schizophrenic Psychosis by Direct Analytic Therapy," *Psychiatric Quarterly,* Vol. 21, January, 1947.
"Method of Resolving Acute Catatonic Excitement," *Psychiatric Quarterly,* Vol. 20, April, 1946.

SULLIVAN, HARRY STACK
Conceptions of Modern Psychiatry, The William Alanson White Psychiatric Foundation, Washington, D. C., 1947.
"Introduction to the Study of Interpersonal Relations," *Psychiatry,* Vol. I, 1938.
"The Meaning of Anxiety in Psychiatry and in Life," *Psychiatry,* Vol. XI, 1948.

WESTERMARCK, EDVARD
Three Essays on Sex and Marriage, Macmillan and Company, New York, 1934.

INDEX

Milton Keynes UK
Ingram Content Group UK Ltd.
UKHW022105141024
449569UK00031B/1791